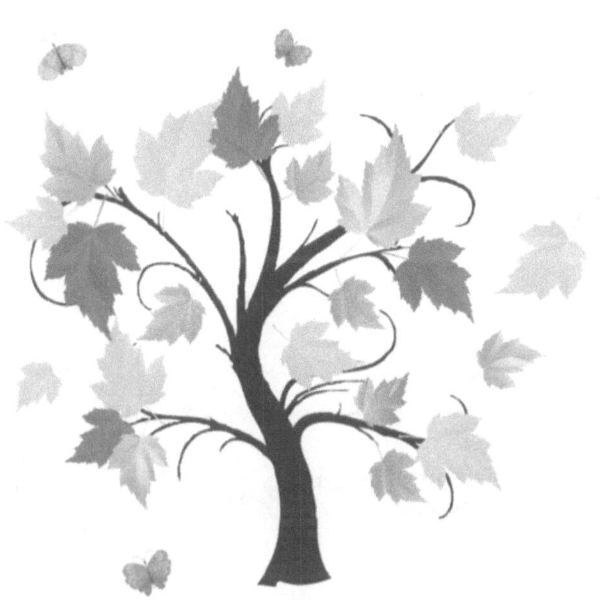

AN INSIDER'S VIEW OF

Emotional Traumas

HOW TO HELP OR SEEK HELP

DINESH KUMAR

ISBN 978-93-81836-85-9
© Dinesh Kumar 2014
Cover Design: Qualcom Designs
Layouts: Ajay Shah
Printing: Repro India Ltd

Published in India 2014 by
BODY & SOUL BOOKS
An imprint of
LEADSTART PUBLISHING PVT LTD
Trade Centre, Level 1, Bandra Kurla Complex
Bandra (E), Mumbai 400 051, INDIA
T + 91 22 40700804 **F** +91 22 40700800
E info@leadstartcorp.com
W www.leadstartcorp.com
US Office Axis Corp, 7845 E Oakbrook Circle, Madison, WI 53717, USA

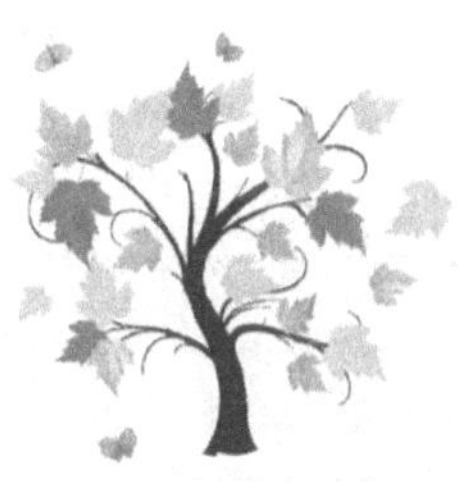

To All Counsellors,
many of whom provide free
counselling services at their centres.
And above all,
to my counsellor-wife Jaya,
whose inputs added great value to the book.

DINESH KUMAR has been a mental health counsellor for 20 years. He has handled a wide spectrum of cases including depression, anxiety, stress, suicidal inclinations, low self-esteem, as well as adolescent and marital issues. Dinesh co-founded a counselling centre in Bangalore, which currently has 30 counsellors, and provides free counselling to clients of widely varying ages and backgrounds.

What drew him to this field? Four decades ago, he went through a long and disturbing personal experience with depression and suicidal thoughts. In the absence of professional help, and with the social stigma attached to such issues, he suffered through that avoidable mental anguish – alone. Through sheer persistence and will power, he moved to a state of positivity. Many years later, he heard of an organization that trained lay counsellors, and so entered the domain. His aim is to let people know they do not have to suffer alone, the way he did; and to move them from a state of helplessness to one of hopefulness. Few people know that the majority of emotional disturbances can be resolved with guidance from a lay counsellor; only extreme cases need referral to a specialist.

Dinesh says: *Those who seek counselling are brave – no one has to suffer alone. Show me a person who claims not to have undergone stress, mild depression, anxiety or marital problems, and I will show you a liar. These may be transient, but affect us all... When does one need counselling? When these conditions become overwhelming and begin to take a toll on our full potential... There are stigmas/ myths attached to mental health; this book seeks to clarify/demystify the subject in a conversational, easy-to-understand style.*

Dinesh has worked with the Indian Air Force, as well as in the corporate world, which gave him an extensive engagement with people and situations. He feels that staying in touch with young people, who continually question and challenge one's beliefs, keeps one connected to the current context of life. A passionate runner, even at 76, Dinesh participates in marathons in India and abroad. His articles have appeared in leading newspapers. He has also authored the book, *Corporate Capers.* Dinesh can be reached at: deejayjogs@gmail.com

CONTENTS

Introduction...7
A Brief History of Psychotherapy.............................10

PART I: Cases & Consequences..............................12
When a suicidal person calls 13
All I want is a fair boy 28
All it needed was a pinch of tobacco.......................44
From one bed to another..55
Put some sense into this boy's head 63
This one ended in divorce 73
A case of seasickness 83
In love, but cannot make love................................. 91
It is time to stop playing 100
Yes darling, no darling, hello darling 106
From victim to victor..115
What will people say? 121
Having his cake and eating it too..........................126

PART II: Spreadsheet of Mental Issues 131
Spirituality & counselling: An alternative View 132
Are you living in an abusive marriage? 135
How is your marriage going? 138
Problem child? Not really.......................................141
Cry of a counsellor...144
Dealing with low self-esteem.................................147
Marital music..150
Primal wounds 152
The sceptre of anxiety 154
The whys of divorce..157
When deep in love: do not marry...........................160
Choose happiness 163

Contents

Sharing Grief 168
Child sexual abuse & the aftermath 170
Mental health indicators 173
Ethics of counsellors 176

PART III: Mental Conditions: an overview 180

Empathy, the Power Within 189

Conclusion 190

Select List Of Counselling Centres 191

Suggested Reading for Counsellors 193

Acknowledgements 194

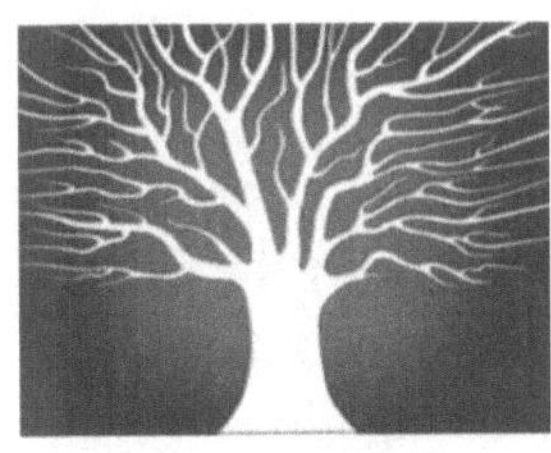

A minimally trained lay therapist who exercises a great capacity to love, will achieve psycho-therapeutic results that equal those of the very best psychiatrists. ~ M Scott Peck, author of *The Road Less Travelled.*

I begin this book with this quotation from my guru in psychotherapy – Dr. M Scott Peck. I have studied and practised therapy for two decades, and in this pursuit, I have learnt much from the leading lights in the field of mental health – people like William Glasser, the proponent of Reality Therapy, and Carl R Rogers, whose philosophy of a client-centred, non-directive and non-judgmental approach, is the backbone of my counselling practice. I have also gained from what Robert Carkhuff and JM Fuster have written. Any aspiring counsellor ought to keep in his library two books, written in simple language, by Father Joe Currie – books from which originated the concept of lay counselling. These are: *The Barefoot Counsellor* and *In The Path Of The Barefoot Counsellor.* But if I were to name one guru as the guiding beacon of my profession, it is Dr M Scott Peck. The reason for this partiality is that Dr Peck combines psychotherapy with love, traditional values, and spiritual growth. I believe – after reading his works and having seen it in many of the cases I have handled – that results are sometimes achieved by the grace of God. He also makes a strong case for moving away from a cut-and-dried approach to therapy and including the 'miracle of serendipity.

This volume is mainly directed towards counsellors – both the beginners as well as the experienced. My personal view is that no matter how experienced we become, there are always new insights to be gained from the literature connected with the subject. I have read some books repeatedly, at intervals, and found new learning with each reading. I believe our understanding develops as we evolve during our own life.

Additionally, the attempt here is to create awareness in the general public about mental health issues and to inform about ways in which to seek help when needed, instead of suffering alone. Family and friends of people dealing with mental health issues, will also learn how to be more effective caregivers. The idea has been to write this book in a simple and straightforward way, devoid of the technical jargon that specialists tend to use. It is also an attempt to counterbalance information overload about our physical health – from bust-to-hip ratios and BMI, calories burnt per hour of exercise or during seven-minutes of sex in bed. That there should be such over-leveraging of physical health issues when depression will soon be the world's biggest killer, is something to ponder over. Do we need to know more about the effects of wearing high heels when suicides and divorce rates are galloping? When it comes to mental health, the general perception is either yes or no – either you are sane or a nutcase; you are fine or need to be in a psychiatric ward. It is rarely understood that much like physical sprains, there are transient mental sprains or disturbances that can be healed with the help of a trained counsellor. This is true the world over. The idea of these pages is to bring these issues out into the open and remove the stigma attached to mental health.

I believe this book will be useful to another segment of readership – students of psychology – who study theory of the mind in classroom settings but lose out on the application of that knowledge in real life situations. This became repeatedly clear to me when some psychology students attended the counselling courses at which I participated as faculty. One of the statements they made, said it all: My God, I didn't know *this* is what counselling is about!

Confidentiality is a non-negotiable principle to which all therapists adhere to. In the case descriptions used here, names have been changed

Introduction

and particulars suitably disguised to preserve anonymity. In some cases, two or more client issues have been clubbed together to highlight important points. Also, since some cases are resolved in weeks while others take more than a year, I have retained only the highlights. The terms *counselling* and *therapy* are used interchangeably, and for this I seek the pardon of the purists. Strictly speaking, a *therapist* is formally trained, but a *counsellor* does not necessarily hold a diploma/degree in the subject.

It is important to state here unequivocally that entering psychotherapy is an act of courage, not weakness, as many believe. Brave are they who say to themselves: This issue I am dealing with needs resolution. I have tried by myself but have not succeeded. I need professional help, just as I would if I were dealing with diabetes.

The return on time invested by a counsellor comes in many forms, but the most important is the realization after each case, that the client *is free from this issue at this point of time.* A counsellor also faces repeated reminders that it could be him sitting in the client's chair. I strongly believe in the dictum: If *you* know the *why* of the subject, you will know the *how* of it – that is, how to apply the knowledge gained. And therefore, at the end of each chapter, there is an addendum titled *Guruspeak*, which gives readers additional inputs I have culled from my reading of the works written by experts in the field.

***

ED NOTE: 'He' has been used throughout in a gender-neutral manner.

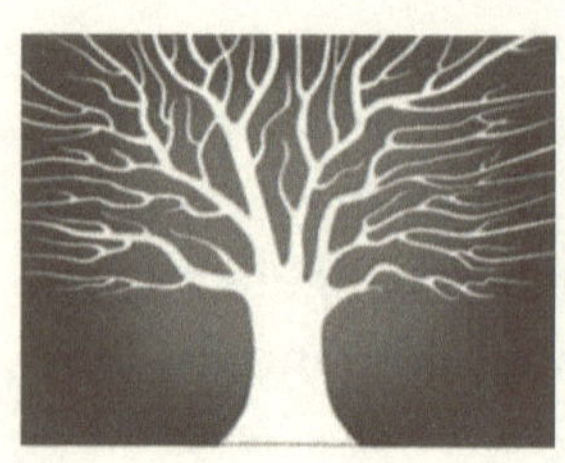

Before we deal with the case studies that will give readers insights into the process of counselling, here is a very brief history of psychotherapy, to provide a context to counselling. Anyone with a passing knowledge of psychology will have heard of Sigmund Freud, the Austrian who is regarded as the founder of psychoanalysis, which for him meant exploring the unconscious mind. He believed that his mental patients struggled to adjust to their environment and so developed faulty thinking and behaviour. Their behaviour gave him clues to the problems/causes underlying their symptoms. Understanding this struggle brought him closer to his patients. As therapists and counsellors, we are not expected to label the struggle, only to observe and understand.

Other pioneers followed Freud. One name that stands out is Carl Rogers. He started client-centred therapy, requiring therapists to be non-judgmental and non-directive. His idea was that counselling provided self-generated insights to grapple with the issues clients faced, and which lie unperceived because the person is deeply enmeshed in the struggle. Carkuff carried this concept further, saying that once the insight is picked up by the client, the counsellor should co-travel with him to outline an action plan, and support him till he is well established on the new course.

M Scott Peck wrote: *Life is difficult and we need discipline to solve life's problems. Without discipline we can solve nothing. With some discipline we can solve some of the problems. With total discipline, we can solve all problems.* He added that problems were the cutting edge that distinguished success from failure. Problems call forth our wisdom and courage.

A Brief History of Psychotherapy

He further added that the period of intensive therapy is a period of intensive growth, in which the client may undergo more changes than some people experience in a lifetime. For this growth spurt to occur, a proportionate amount of the 'old self' must be given up. In fact, the process of 'giving up' usually begins with the first session with the counsellor.

In the mid-60s, however, doubters appeared on the scene, who rubbished the whole concept of counselling. Massive research followed with the consensus emerging that psychotherapy provided a great deal of help and relief in about 80% of cases. In the remaining 20%, failure to help could be attributed to the therapist's incompetence or the client's weak desire to effect change. Counselling is now established worldwide. In India, it stands at the threshold of change and acceptance.

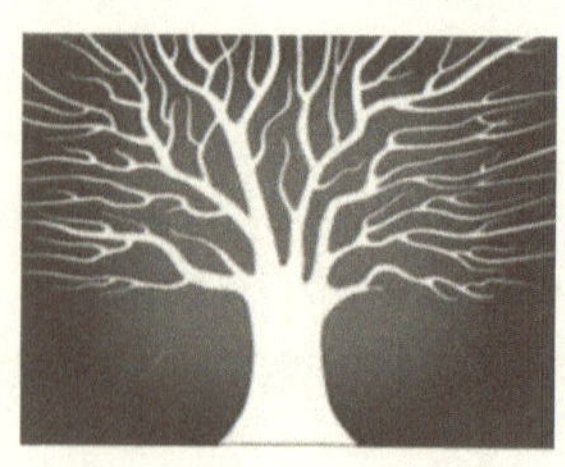

Part I: CASES & CONSEQUENCES

This part of the book presents typical cases that counsellors deal with in their professional lives. The intention here is to give an insider's view of counselling, and bring into the open various emotional issues that most of us deal with. How well we handle these issues depends on the coping mechanisms we build on a day-to-day basis. Some people are able to surmount the issues whereas others become submerged and overwhelmed by them, and need counselling.

Most of this work is done at counselling centres located in the major cities, but they are woefully few in number. There is a crying need to build a counselling infrastructure on a massive scale if we are to cope with the stresses modern-day society is experiencing. The majority of counselling centres are run by non-profit organisations and have volunteers on their rolls. One does not have to seek an appointment and most do not even charge a fee for services rendered. A senior counsellor conducts what is called a screening session, to establish the nature of the issue/s the person is dealing with, and then allots a counsellor relevant to his needs. Usually, the sessions are held on a weekly basis and the duration is approximately an hour. If required, the frequency and the duration is altered.

It needs to be stated here, over and over again, that *brave are they who say to themselves: I will not suffer alone. I will step out, seek help, and live to my true potential.*

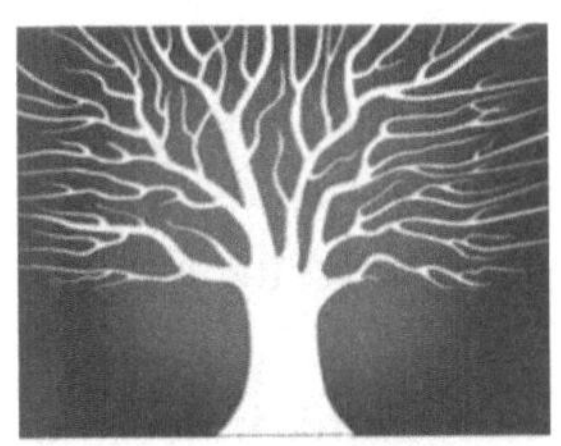

Suicide is a permanent solution to a temporary problem. ~ Phil Donahue

Suicide is defined as an act to voluntarily end one's life. But let me start with a real life episode which had a happy ending. Today, Rashmi is a highly successful team leader in an InfoTech company. But eight years ago, she was facing the trauma of a failed suicide attempt. Let us go back to the beginning.

A couple in their fifties came to see me without prior appointment. It was an emergency, they said; their sixteen-year-old daughter had attempted to commit suicide. On that day, her younger brother, impatient that Rashmi had taken far too long in the toilet, knocked on the door (as younger brothers are wont to do). There was no reply. He alerted their parents and all three of them pushed the door open to find Rashmi lying on the floor, bleeding profusely from a deep cut in her right wrist. They quickly bandaged the wrist and lifted her onto her bed. Rashmi was hurting, but still able to talk. According to her parents, she kept saying: "Why did you save me? I don't want to live anymore. I want to die. Let me go."

Her mother helped her through the day. Neither parent wanted to take Rashmi to hospital lest the failed suicide attempt become known and reach the press. They sedated her and let her sleep. The next morning, they drove her to my office. When I asked them what could have led her to such a desperate action, both parents were unable to give any reason. The father made an insensitive comment: "I don't know whether it was to draw attention to herself that Rashmi did what she did." They said she had been chirpy and jovial when she got up that morning. Her brother had teased her and she had responded in full measure. It had come as a shock to them both. "We just don't know what happened and thought we should bring her to you for a consultation," they said. The thrust of their request was that I do what I could to drill some sense into Rashmi's head; and not to tell anyone about the incident.

Following that brief interview, I went out to see Rashmi, in another room. I softly asked her, "Rashmi, what happened?" Rashmi wept profusely. The only sentence that came from her lips was, "I don't want to live; I just don't want to live." She kept repeating the same statement while looking down and crying. I called the receptionist to hold Rashmi's hands and rub her back, to help her let go of her deeply embedded emotions. But she kept crying and repeating, "I have had enough. I don't want to live. I just don't want to live. I don't know why I was so unlucky that my brother noticed my absence. I am so unlucky, I am so unlucky, I am so unlucky!"

The rest of the session was spent in tears, cursing her luck. No coherent reason for her behaviour came through. I repeatedly I told her that I knew she must have been going through hell to decide to take such an extreme step. "Life was just not worth living for you Rashmi," I said. She nodded. "The pain was so great that you wanted to end it all, Rashmi." She nodded again and sobbed. "You just could not see any light at the end of the tunnel Rashmi, and felt you couldn't carry on." She kept nodding at my statements and crying with her face down. But I could see she felt that for once, her anguish had been understood. The nods and slightly less tense body gave me that feedback.

I then told Rashmi that there was no one who could take away her right to do what she wanted with her life. I slipped in a remark that whether she wanted to live or not was her choice but suicide was an extreme and final step. I asked her to promise me that she would not do anything like that for one week, just one week, so I could get to know her better. After that, whatever she did was her choice. "Will you give me that promise?" I asked. She nodded. "Let us shake hands on that." I extended my hand and she held out her hand. My secretary, who was present, said spontaneously, "Not fair – I too, want that promise. I too, want to shake Rashmi's hand." Rashmi smiled just a wee bit and held out her hand again.

I gave Rashmi my mobile number and told her that if she was in distress or had any suicidal thoughts, she was free to call me to chat at any time of day or night. In fact, I would be most disappointed if she did not, if such a need arose. There was the suggestion of a smile on her face as we made an appointment for the next day.

I went back to where the parents were waiting anxiously. I told them that no attempted suicide is done to draw attention and there was nothing like a fake call. Advising them to be gentle with her and let her decide at her own pace, I cautioned them against getting into a strong advisory, well-meaning mode: 'We will always be there for you...', 'Your parents will do anything for you...' etc. No questioning either: 'Why did you take this silly step?' 'Why didn't you talk to us?' I also told them that nothing they said at this time would make any sense to her. "Just be there with her and engage with her at the level she chooses to engage in. Do not try to create a 'cheer-up' atmosphere to buck her up. It will produce exactly opposite results to what you think. Just be there. She needs your presence at this stage and not your sermons."

Important Issues about Suicide Cases

This may be the right time to talk about a few issues connected with suicide cases. The most important of all is that in suicide there are no 'fake calls'. Each call has to be taken seriously. It may well be that some attempts are of lower intensity and consequent harm, but you will never know which ones those are. It is a fact in psychology, that people who have failed in their initial suicide attempt/s, often repeat it/them and succeed.

The second issue is that people with certain personality defects may make a fake attempt as a form of blackmail or threat, but we are not discussing such personality issues here. How one identifies and deals with such issues is a chapter in itself. But to get back to suicidal tendencies, how often we hear that the person was looking happy and jovial just before the event, just as Rashmi's parents said. It is, in fact, the most dangerous period for a suicidal person because, having given out many hints, s/he then gives up as no one seems to be listening, and masks their true, depressive feelings by seeming to be energetic and happy. In some cases, they become tranquil and calm. Nothing better describes the mask suicidal people wear than this Urdu couplet, sung by the late gazal maestro, Jagjit Singh: *Tum itna kyon muskara rahe ho, kya gham hai jis ko chhupa rahe ho* [Why are you smiling so? What is that sadness you are trying to hide?]

Suicide is an act of violence, and violence against the self (like any violence), needs high energy. In fact, a suicidal person is both weak and strong – vulnerable in their feelings of total hopelessness; and strong in committing the final act. Another fact of suicide is that in most cases the person gives strong indications or signals which cry out for our attention. However, since most of us are not trained to pick up those signals and our receivers are not tuned to the victim's transmitters, we miss out on these desperate messages. 'I don't see any light at the end of the tunnel...', 'Frankly, I am fed up with this kind of living...', 'Nothing seems to work for me....', 'No one seems to care...', 'I really don't know what to do...', 'I am a failure...', 'Whatever I do, I end up in a mess...', are some statements that should alert us that all is not well. And sometimes direct statements like, 'I think the time has come to end my life and get out of this mess'. And on the rare occasions we may pick up the signal, our responses (often from goodwill but sheer ignorance), push the person closer to suicide.

IGNORANT RESPONSES

- 'Don't be silly. Your whole life is in front of you. Why are you entertaining such silly thoughts?'
- 'Buck up! What is your problem? I went through a much bigger mess with my boyfriend. Your problem is nowhere near mine.'

- 'Let's go to a movie and get this silly idea out of your head.'
- 'Go for a walk in the park; you will feel better.'
- 'Here, have a cup of coffee; you will feel better.'

The last was what one well intentioned mother did in a real life case. The daughter had poured her heart out and almost said as directly as she could, that she was going to end her life. The mother responded saying she would go and make some coffee to help her relax. While making the coffee, she heard a bullet shot. The daughter had picked up her father's loaded pistol and shot herself.

A Victim's Thoughts

The suicidal person who receives sermons, thinks like this: 'You are talking about yourself and your boyfriend. Dash it! I am talking about myself. As if I have not already tried to divert my attention from my thoughts by seeing a movie. I have tried every darn thing but I am still in this horrible mess.' These are the thoughts that go through the mind of a desperate person who is hiding his desperation behind a mask of happiness.

Recommended Approach

If these are not the right approaches, what are? Clearly, it is to relate at the feeling-and-thought level of the person in question. Paraphrasing the statements of the suicidal is not only useful but very important.

- 'So what you feel is that life is too much of a burden to carry.'
- 'What you are saying is that despite trying everything, you can't seem to find a solution.'
- You feel the pain of living is too much to bear.'

Remember that people who commit suicide are those who consider the pain of living to be more than the pain of dying. That is the depth of their distress. Body language is important as well. Lean forward and give your full attention to the person; respond at the same level of energy the person is displaying.

This one will come as a shocker: Bringing the subject of suicide into the open. Use the S word and ask whether the person is feeling like committing suicide. Most people believe that by saying it, we are putting the idea into the person's mind. Psychology looks at it very differently. If the thought is already present and fermenting, the issue will come out into the open instead of festering in a tormented mind. And if the thought is not there, it will be vigorously rebuffed: 'No way! I have no such thought' or 'No, I am not that desperate'. In therapy sessions, counsellors often use the approach of asking about suicide directly in the very first session – to know what the situation really is.

SUBSEQUENT SESSIONS

Rashmi came back the next evening, looking slightly better. I welcomed her with the compliment that her sense of punctuality was commendable (compliments, if genuine, help in such cases of low self-esteem – when the person thinks that their life is not worth living. On the other hand, an insincere compliment informs the receiver it is worthless). In counselling terms, we call such sincere compliments *positive strokes*.

The mother sat outside while I spoke with Rashmi. In the case of young people, I try to make my sessions chatty, speaking the language they speak, lest they get overawed by my age and position. Over the next few sessions with Rashmi, what emerged was a typical case of rejection from childhood onwards. She told me her elder sister was the queen and she the equivalent of a maid. All her childhood she had heard: 'Look at your sister, she is so smart and hard working and look at you.' 'Look at your sister, she is so confident, so well groomed, and look at you.' 'Look at your sister, she's is always in the first three ranks and you are always hitting the bottom of the class.' 'Look at your sister, she takes care of guests when they drop in and look at you, you go and hide yourself in your room and we have to come and pull you out.'

This was the core of her life described variously on different days, using different examples. The more she talked about her life, the less frequent became her crying. But just as I would begin to feel she was on the upward path, she would revert to square one and think seriously of suicide again. This may be the time to mention that this case took 50 sessions before I began weaning her from weekly to fortnightly to monthly appointments, to ultimately letting her fly on her own wings.

Coming back to her suicide attempt – the trigger was her music teacher, who was preparing the class for a live performance. One evening, the teacher assembled the girls and said that she would be picking the five best for the live performance. Rashmi was told she was not in consideration and thrown out of the group with the cruel remark: 'I don't know why I have been wasting my time and energy on you. You have no talent. I suggest you stop coming. There is no need for your parents to waste their money on you.' The following morning she made the attempt on herself.

In all these sessions, I concentrated on her strong points, like her helpful nature, that she minded her own business, her interest in baking, and the beautiful crochet work she did. It worked for a while and then, she would break down in self-pity and self-condemnation again. Again her life would not be worth living. After about five months, she began to regard me, I suspect, as her missing father, the kind of father she would have loved to have. This is a common phenomenon, known as transference in counselling. Transference is the image of perceptions one develops in childhood.

After five months I came to the conclusion that while Rashmi was making progress, her fall backs were still too frequent. At this stage, I decided to use the 'hurt to heal' approach. For the well-being of the client, out of love and support, counsellors sometimes use this method. However, it is something I use only as a last resort.

I began telling her that I believed she was enjoying the attention she was getting from me week after week. One hour of total attention had become her need. This is something that can happen with people with low self-esteem. She would protest, cry, and talk about her parents and friends being nasty. I told her firmly that she should not mention anyone, her parents, friends or family, because they were not present in the counselling room. Since they were not present, there was nothing we could do about them. I gave her insights to clarify that if she was waiting for the behaviour of others to change, she was playing a loser's game, and it was a waste of time. While this approach worked for a couple of weeks, she would soon fall back into the blame game, holding the world responsible for her misery.

When one has worked with the client for months, one develops a conversational approach, hoping to provide some insights for the client to work on. In one session, I told Rashmi that she was being a lazy person: "You want to take the easy course. When people criticize you, you hide and blame others for being cruel. Have you succeeded in changing even one person? If the answer is 'no', then you will have to think of something else. If you continue to travel on the same track, you will keep reaching the same sad station you have visited in the past." She would respond by saying that I did not know what she was going through or had gone through.

In another session, I told her that if she continued in the same way, then I would not have much more to offer. She pleaded with me to continue counselling her. In later sessions I told her that she was living her life according to a script written by others – her parents, teachers and friends: "Do you see that you have made yourself a puppet to so many puppeteers, who pull the strings and you dance?" I also asked her if, even assuming her mother changed, she would spend the rest of her life trying to change her father, her friends and her teacher? "Change your script and tell those who call you no good to shut up and mind their own business. They won't know how to react because they are so used to your being a cry baby." She would contest what I said but deep inside she knew that for others to change, she had to change herself.

All I was doing was making Rashmi realize that she had to learn to face the facts of life and not run away and seek shelter. Ultimately, what worked for her was when I asked her to number all the people to whom she had given the power of her life. "Take it back," I said, "and take it back now." It took many months for her to start thinking well of herself. After gradually weaning her from counselling, I let the Rashmi bird fly.

Mission of the Counsellor

The counsellor's aim is to try to help the client to run his/her life independently at the end of the counselling sessions. Often, clients become too dependent and hooked to having regular meetings to manage their life on a day-to-day basis. In some ways, the counsellor becomes a crutch for the client, somewhat like the bottle becomes a strong need for an alcoholic. This, in counselling terms, is called co-dependency. The client starts getting dressed up to meet the counsellor on the appointed day as if s/he is going to a social meeting. Counsellors are aware of this and therefore gradually reduce the number of visits from weekly to fortnightly to monthly, and then conclude the contract with the clear message that if the client ever needs to return, help would be available. The main aim of the counsellor is to move the client from a state of dependency to one of independence. Only after the person has tasted independence can s/he enter the world of interdependence – a state where all crutches have been discarded.

Rashmi still calls me. She often mentions how yet another man in her life has taken advantage of her. Her self-esteem is still not fully built to be able to run life on a win-win basis. She still is in a lose-win status in many situations. However, from being on the verge of suicide to functioning as an IT person in a prestigious company, has been a long and arduous journey of personal growth for her.

Transference & Counter-Transference

Earlier, I used the terms 'transference' and (its opposite) counter-transference. Transference is one of Freud's greatest insights into psychotherapy. He observed that though he was physically no great looker, many clients were attracted to him. He studied the phenomenon and concluded that many childhood conflicts and assumptions get transferred to the client's current relationship with the counsellor/ analyst. 'He is like the father I always wanted.' 'I wish my husband was someone like him.' 'He is such an understanding person.' These are some indicators of transference of feelings from client to counsellor. Transference frequently happens when people are under stress. In marital counselling in particular, transference is very common. The counsellor is seen as someone who fills a vacuum.

As an aside, it is believed that psycho-therapists are more prone to falling into extra-marital relationships than other professionals. Counsellors need to be aware of the transference that may be taking place in the minds of their clients. It is also believed that transference can cause a bias in the mind of the counsellor and bring in a judgmental approach to the process. My view is that if transference works for the benefit of the client, it is well used. If Rashmi saw in me the kind of father she wished she had and was willing to take my inputs, I saw no harm in it. If, on the other hand, in marital counselling, a woman sees me as a romantic substitute and I start taking her side and becoming impatient with the husband, then transference is harmful.

Counter-transference is a phenomenon exactly the opposite of transference. Here the counsellor/therapist starts seeing the client as that missing person – the beautiful wife he always wanted or the understanding husband she wished she had. In such a case, the counsellor/therapist carries a sense of guilt in his mind and starts getting impatient or ignoring the client. Counter-transference can lead to a strong attraction or revulsion to the client. Seeing a person who has, say, evil designs towards others, can lead to repulsive transference and become a source of interference in the process of counselling. Here the counsellor has to beware of emotional involvement. The Achilles heel of an immature therapist is his/her determination to change people at all costs, and they frequently blunder.

When a Suicidal Person Calls, Listen

Some Facts about Suicide

In the time you take to turn a couple of pages of this book, someone somewhere in India will have committed suicide. These are the reported cases but what about those cases that go unreported because of the shame involved with the act? There are many more failed than successful attempts of suicide. A little known fact is that India is one of the few countries which holds a failed attempt to end one's life to be a criminal offence. It is like telling the person: 'You thought you were clever and could end your pain by killing yourself. But you did not know we were watching you. Now we will show you what real pain is.' This is one of the many archaic laws that need to be scrapped unless we wish to remain in the company of those backward nations that still have attempted suicide as an offence on their statute books. The most vulnerable are adolescents and old people. Also, women try to commit suicide more often than men, but succeed less frequently.

Myths about Suicide

There are some myths about the subject that we need to put on the table. The first is that people attempt suicide to draw attention to themselves and that often these attempts are fake. It needs to be stated clearly and emphatically that there are no fake calls and even if there are, do we know which ones fall into the fake category? Therefore, all such attempts have to be taken seriously. The second point is that those who have failed in their attempt, continue to try because the thought of ending life does not vanish with a failed attempt. Those who try to commit suicide are serious about their mission. Through this final act, they also want to show defiance and prove to the world that they are in charge of their life and they can do what they want with it.

Some triggers for attempted suicide are listed below:
- Arguments with parents or between parents
- Loss of parents
- Divorce of parents
- Break-up of a relationship
- Failing grades

When a Suicidal Person Calls, Listen

- Loss of a job
- Loss of face
- Boredom
- Low self-esteem
- Stress
- A series of suicides impel some to consider the act
- Helplessness or hopelessness
- Illness
- Depression
- Alcoholism.

What comes next is very important: The usual response from well intentioned people that with time things will work out, *does not make any sense to the person planning suicide.* Never challenge the reality of such a person, because their thoughts and feelings are real to them. Remember, we can neither cajole people out of their intentions nor distract them from their thoughts. Jollying or sermonizing, are the last things we should do. Just be there and encourage the person to share their thoughts and feelings.

Problems never exist in a pure state;
there is always a human being attached to them.

GURUSPEAK

Let us remember that the common emotion involved in suicide is hopelessness-helplessness, and the internal attitude of the person is that of ambivalence. The person feels constricted because s/he feels unendurable psychological pain. Suicide can strike anyone, any family, at any age, and each suicidal person is unique.

Often we believe there are those who fall in the category of 'suicidal type'. But that is just another among the many other myths. And therefore it is difficult to predict, identify, assess and prevent suicides. Some other myths include believing suicide is an irrational act. It is not. It is an act that has been rationalized in the mind of the person and s/he really wants to die. I have heard people call those who commit suicide insane. There are also those amongst us who think the act of self-destruction is inherited or a genetic predilection. Others believe children do not commit suicide. *All these assumptions are simply not true.*

One of the signs or indicators that suicidal persons exhibit is that they begin to gift away possessions that are dear to them. It has been mentioned earlier that perceiving and understanding the feelings of the client is very important to the process of counselling. We have to look for loaded words, for they are a measure of the intensity or gravity of the issue the person is facing or feeling. The emotional range of the suicidal personality is extensive. They generally feel trapped, frightened, hopeless, distressed, lonely, worthless, depressed and confused. You will see signs of boredom, hostility, shame and anger in them.

One of the major tasks of the counsellor is to keep watch on the level and intensity of the client's lethal intent and try and steer the person away from negative thoughts to the positive aspects of their life and personality. The idea is to reveal and focus on the very issues which offer concrete reasons to celebrate his life. There is none amongst us who does not have at least a few bright spots and silver linings. Unfortunately, it is the inner critic within the suicidally inclined, who overwhelms and overshadows the good things, by insistently saying we are no good and hence unworthy of life.

One important function counsellors have to perform is to counsel caregivers like parents and siblings, about how to deal with daily issues while the process of counselling is going on. A counsellor meets the client for an hour or two on a weekly basis but the rest of the time is spent in the family setting. The family needs to stay calm and not discuss the issue with friends and family because the load of free advice will confuse rather than help them. In case there are doubts or queries, the family should seek clarifications from the counsellor and coordinate on how to build their coping skills. Both caregivers and counsellors have to remember not to either over-react or under-react in dealing with suicidal cases. I mention this because I have observed both these tendencies in many people I have met in such circumstances. The sage advice of Eugene Kennedy and Sarah Charles is that if one is to understand the mindset of the suicidal person, then it is important to see things from his point of view, which means everything looks black and bleak.

The most common causes leading to suicide have already been listed but there are many others that merit mention here. Painful injuries, extreme loneliness, continued dependence on others, legal issues, school-related problems, alcohol abuse, terminal illnesses without remission, and severe stress, are some other reasons which lead people to take the extreme step of taking their life. Others may take the decision because their lives have become dependent on others for their daily living and they are unhappy with this condition of perpetual dependency.

One of the most important contributions a counsellor can make is to make clients talk about those few things that work in their lives. An expert puts it this way: 'You say that there are lots of things you like about life and there are reasons for, as well as against, staying alive. Can you tell me more about these?' The idea clearly is to move the person away from a state of perpetual negativity to one of positivity; to let the person see some ray of light at the end of the tunnel.

We should always bear in mind that the greatest risk of suicide is when the person is alone and has an opportunity. A non-invasive, watchful eye is very important until the healing process has taken place. Therefore it is also important to keep those you trust, in the loop about what is going on, without encouraging overreaction or panic. The last thing you want is to start an intellectual conversation with the suicidal person on the pros and cons of committing suicide along the following lines: 'Have you ever thought of what others will think of your family if you were to take such a drastic step?' Or 'Have you considered that no one will offer a proposal of marriage for your younger sister because of the stigma attached to your suicide?' *No, please…definitely no.*

The rehabilitation of such a person and their transition to a wholesome life, takes a long time, even when the risk has been minimized. One of the sure signs of progress is when the person starts saying words to the effect: 'I can't believe I even considered ending my life for a stupid reason like that….' Until then, a better-safe-than-sorry approach is recommended. Quite simply, it translates into unconditional support, love, empathy and doing everything to boost the self-image/esteem of the person. Encouraging him to keep a diary, recording thoughts and feelings as they come and go, is another important tool for venting. If done at the end of the day, it relaxes the stressed mind. For most people, the time after sunset, particularly in winter, is difficult to handle.

Perhaps the most important thing to mention here from the counsellor's perspective, is that if the client decides to harm himself, do not have any guilt feelings about it for we know, if a person is determined to end his life, he *will* succeed, despite our best efforts to stop him.

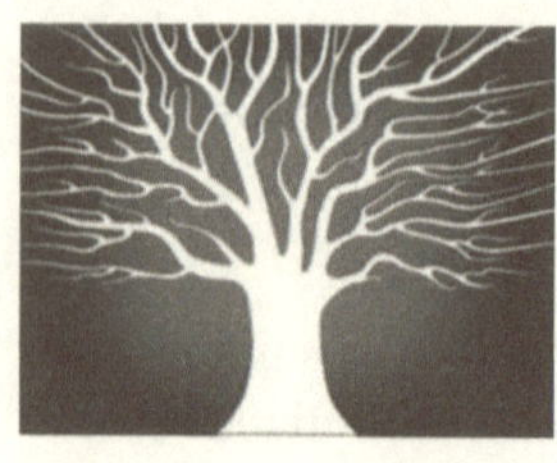

I loathe narcissism, but I approve of vanity. ~ Diana Vreeland

Rani and her daughter Roopa, walked into my counselling chamber with their heads down, not sure whether they were doing the right thing in meeting me. Of the two, Roopa, going by her body language, looked more distraught and downcast. They sat down tentatively, looking at each other, not knowing where to start. Having experienced this in the past, I kept my counsel and let them take their own time. Counselling has taught me to be comfortable with silences. Often, the silences of a client tells us more than his spoken words. We can get in touch with his feelings, and that is a very important feedback in this profession. The idea is to let the conversation flow at the chosen pace of the counselee and not rush in to break the silence or compress the process. Doing that stifles the ventilation process of the caller. The pace of conversation, particularly in the initial phases, has to be determined by the caller.

Rani said that she did not know where to start. I encouraged her to say the first thing that came into her mind. In a voice barely above a whisper, she told me she had two daughters. The older one had married and moved to the US, where she now lived with her husband and two children. Roopa was the other child. She had just graduated and was aspiring to be a management graduate from an overseas university. Roopa had fallen in love with a boy from a different caste and lower economic strata and that was when all the problems started. A fairly functional family had become totally dysfunctional and the relationship between Roopa's parents, and between father and daughter, lay in tatters.

All I want is a Fair Boy

Roopa was on the verge of an emotional breakdown. I knew she was suppressing her sobs and I saw that her body was wrapped in tension. One gentle touch by me on her knee and she began crying… and crying. Between sobs, she said: "I don't want to live. I just don't want to live. This is too much." After a few sips of water and letting go some part of her sadness, she regained her composure and sat with her shoulders drooping, her eyes fixed on the ground.

The mother began the narrative, giving the gist of what had been happening in their lives. What she said was enough for me to know the context and reflect over the issue. Reflection on inputs is an important part of counselling. This is what she had to say: They lived in a bungalow in an up-market locality and had ("by the grace of God"), a comfortable life. Her husband was a first generation entrepreneur who, by sheer hard work, had set up a growing business, manufacturing engineering components and most of what the company produced was exported to Europe. The business left her husband drained, exhausted, and stressed at the end of the day. He needed someone from the family to assist him and finally take over. She was also anxious because her husband had had a mild heart attack some years ago and was on medication.

Their son-in-law was persuaded to shift back to India, but within a year he decided to return to the US, not being able to cope with his father-in-law's authoritative behaviour, coupled with a very different living and working environment. He chose a hard-working life in the US over the cushy life of comfort offered to him in India. The factory was being run by Rani's husband with the help of a long-term, loyal manager. But who would support and eventually succeed him in the business was a subject of perpetual discussion. Rani said her husband would rant and rave about who would take over the industrial empire he had built from scratch, declaring: "I can't see my hard work and sweat go to waste. I shall not allow it. I shall not."

All I want is a Fair Boy

I told the mother and daughter that I needed to see them separately in the subsequent session, and assured them that every word they uttered would be in total confidence and nobody would get a whiff of it. The entire conversation during this and following sessions, I assured them, would be treated with the respect and confidentiality a therapeutic relationship between counsellor and counselee deserved.

There are more assurances that are necessary for the therapist to give to distressed counselees but it is better to give it to them in small digestible doses. But the confidentiality factor is uppermost in the minds of those who come for therapy. Sometimes, to allay any doubts in the minds of counselees, I tell them that if I see them outside my counselling chamber, I will not recognize them, unless they chose to recognize me. I walked to the gate of the building with my arm resting gently on the shoulder of the young suffering girl, to build a rapport with her. Rapport and trust are most necessary in forging a therapeutic relationship between counsellor and counselee.

ABOUT COUNSELLING

A few words on the subject of counselling may be of value here for novice counsellors and lay readers who may be clear about the physical aspect of living but remain ignorant about the mental issues and emotional traumas in people's daily lives. For example, what does it mean to live and cope with a deeply depressed person; how to resolve marital issues that crop up in many marriages; how to deal with rebellious adolescents who were so good and obedient until just the other day? Anxiety is every person's burden; depression is everyone's illness; and so are many other issues that relate to the functioning of the mind. Yet, ask anyone about mental health and you will get the impression that most people are vague about it. The kind of response you will get is this: 'Mentally healthy means being sane and mentally unhealthy means being insane, a nut case'.

Most of us are clear about physical fractures and sprains, and where to seek help for them, but we are completely ignorant about mental fractures and mental sprains. We are clear where to go when we have an issue with our eyesight or for any other physical disturbances we experience. B*ut how many of us know that the World Health Organization has declared that depression, not diabetes or heart attacks, is going to be the biggest killer in the future*? Even assuming we have read this statement, the next question that arises is about our knowledge of how to detect signs of depression and where to seek help.

Another point that needs to be mentioned is that *most mental issues are like sprains – transient disturbances that can be resolved by a trained therapist and need no popping of pills or rushing to psychiatrists* (who are too few to tackle the overwhelming range of mental issues of our very large population). The psychiatrist or psychiatric bed-to-patient ratio in India is one of the worst in the whole world. The support system for mental health is woefully inadequate. This is where lay therapists have an invaluable role. Dr. M Scott Peck, a leading American psychiatrist and famous author of the equally famous book, *The Road Less Travelled*, has this to say about lay therapists: *A minimally trained lay therapist who exercises a great capacity to love will achieve psycho-therapeutic results that equal those of the very best psychiatrists.*

Why is there such a dismal situation in our knowledge bank on mental issues? While the media write copiously about every whim and word of an actress – whether worthy of attention or not – no space or time is given to mental health issues which plague a huge percentage of the population. The latest on body mass index (BMI) is regularly featured and extended coverage is gleefully given to various dress malfunctions on the red carpet or at fashion shows. We are treated to photographs of exposed anatomy and within hours we can share in the visual experience of someone's humiliation. This situation is both sad and angry but at the end of the day we have to admit that the only thing in our control is our own responses, and that we cannot take upon ourselves the task of repairing the behaviour of others, least of all the all-powerful media.

All I want is a Fair Boy

Rani and Roopa arrived at the appointed time the following week, and after greeting them, I said I was willing to work with them to resolve the issue; but not to expect instant solutions to a long-festering issue. This disclosure becomes necessary because most people who step in for counselling, come with the impression that the therapist will dispense some kind of to-do list, which once followed, will dissolve the issue/s they are dealing with, rather like an ice pack for sore muscles. Some mental health pundits call it a 'dispensary approach'. I asked the mother to step out to the waiting room while I talked to the daughter for a while. A therapist, in a situation where more than one person is in counselling, has to decide when to see the clients individually and when collectively. That is the therapist's call.

Roopa started hesitantly. This is what she eventually said: "My sister and I had a very comfortable upbringing. We were sent to the best schools. We had everything except that Dad had no time for us. He was so busy that even when he came home, he would be on the phone shouting at someone or the other. Mum had to choose her words carefully while making any suggestion because if he did not like something, he would blow up. Life was in some sort of balance, with mom taking care of us and most of our needs. That is, until I told my mother that I liked a boy from my class and that we were meeting each other after school. I said: "I really like him but don't tell Dad because he will get very angry. It took me some time to tell my mother that the boy was not a Brahmin and that his father was a government officer. That is when my world fell apart. I spent my time hiding and crying all day. My mother insisted I give up these nonsensical thoughts unless I wanted to be thrown out of the house by my Dad. He would never tolerate it. Never, ever. The more I came under pressure, the more I got attracted to Ramesh (the boyfriend), and we would often miss classes since coming home late from classes was totally banned."

What I have narrated here in a few lines, took the pained girl (all of 18 years and five feet three inches), an hour to let me know her story of woe. She cried, sobbed, and stopped, regained her composure, and kept asking me one question repeatedly: "Sir, do you think I have done something wrong? Do you think I have let my parents down?" I told her it was not for me to judge. I was not going through the experience, though I understood her pain. I said I knew what she was feeling – that no one at home was willing to support her and she was left friendless to face this responsibility all on her own. I kept saying I understood her trauma.

A counsellor has to be impartial and not take any position on the emotional issue the client is dealing with. At the same time, it begs clarification that not taking a position or conveying understanding of the situation does not mean agreement. It only means: I understand your pain. In counselling terms, it means empathy, getting under the skin of the person in front of you; understanding their pain and conveying that they have been understood. The counsellor sits in the space of saying to himself: 'If I were in your position, going through the circumstances you are going through, in the environment you live in, if your parents were mine, and the boy you love was my lover, I would be no different than you are now.' This is the level of empathy one has to bring to the counselling chamber.

My therapy guru, M Scott Peck, advises that in much the same way we do not judge the moon, which is covered by a patch of clouds, saying the moon could be much more beautiful if that patch were removed or if it had to be there, it should have been on the lower fringes of the moon, so also we do not judge the client. Empathy means getting under the skin of the client and feeling the feelings the client is experiencing. However, there is one caveat here. We do not judge the person but we certainly judge the act. To give an example: if a person confides that he has stolen something and is dealing with a sense of ongoing guilt, we do not judge the person but that is not to say we do not judge the act of stealing.

EMPATHY/SYMPATHY

Before I go back to the case, we need to understand the difference between empathy and sympathy. The two words are often used interchangeably when they are actually poles apart in meaning. The dissimilarity starts with the origin of the two words. Sympathy is of Greek origin while empathy is German. While sympathizing, we share feelings and grief, relieve burdens and lend a helping hand. While sympathy is a precious virtue in some circumstances, it does not help the other to initiate action. Also, it conveys agreement with the other's feelings. In sympathy, there is emotional involvement. Let me give an example here. Let us say a friend of yours has got divorced recently. While sympathising with her, you might say, 'I really share your pain. This is the last thing your husband should have done to you. You don't deserve this kind of treatment. It is very wrong of your husband to have ditched you at this stage of your life.'

While empathising as a counsellor, you will not take that approach. Empathising would mean: 'I understand your pain of separation. I understand the new responsibilities that you have to take over – the household work, bringing up children and the adjustments of a new life.' Understanding – yes, conveying that understanding – yes, but no taking sides as to whose fault it was that caused the separation.

Sympathy has a strong loyalty factor attached to it, with a how-can-I-let-down-my-friend connotation, but does not help to find a solution. But through empathy, we explore with the client, understand the issue better, try and find a solution, and act. This is very important. In fact, the most important attribute of a counsellor is empathy and hence we need to spend more time on it. To be an empathic person, you have to be a feeling person. You must get in touch with your own feelings before you can feel another's. A high degree of sensitivity is required. You can fake sympathy but you cannot fake empathy.

After the session with Roopa, I called Rani in. She repeated the same story as Roopa but gave some more insights into the context. I asked

All I want is a Fair Boy

her a bit about her life and marriage, not in a probing or inquisitive manner. For a counsellor, probing is not acceptable. Clarifying a situation is different from satisfying one's curiosity. Rani said her husband had provided them with all the material comforts – the best cars for the girls, school, clothes – and that he loved them in his own way. But if there was even the smallest resistance from them or her, he would get very upset. They bought peace by keeping quiet. She had learnt to cope with it but the children had minds of their own. She had tried to persuade Roopa to give up the relationship because she knew it would not work. "It just would not work but she refused to give up. I could not hold it in any longer and told my husband about Roopa falling in love with this boy. From then on, Roopa became an outcaste. She was severely reprimanded and ordered to give up the boy – the idiot ensnaring her to take advantage of their wealth. He told her to stop being foolish and asked repeatedly whether she was willing to leave the boy in exchange for what he had done for her, giving her everything from the day she was born."

I asked how Roopa was handling the situation. Rani began weeping, saying that she could not bear to see her daughter go through this pain. Roopa would lock herself in her room and cry and cry. She ate very little so she had lost a lot of weight in the last few days. "Life at home is simply hell and I don't know what to do. I just don't know," was Rani's constant refrain. She also said she had not shared with Roopa the ultimatum of one month that her father had given, to sort out the mess.

I knew Rani was in a state of hopelessness and I slipped in the thought that what she was facing was one of the many painful realities of life, but that, with some assistance, she would overcome the situation. I knew that at this stage all she needed was hope and I had to give her that. I asked her whether her husband would be willing to meet me, so that I could counsel them as a family. She said she would try but it was not likely because he had often told them they were wasting their time and his money in seeking help. The

All I want is a Fair Boy

mother and daughter then departed for home with heavy hearts but maybe a ray of hope.

THE ABSENT PARTY

In counselling cases, it often happens that one of the parties who is part of the issue, refuses to come. But does that mean the therapist gives up? The answer is clearly no, because the client who is present is the rationale of the therapist's existence and he has no control over those who choose not to accept help. Such situations arise mostly in marital discord cases where one of the partners – usually the husband – does not appear. The absentee party keeps harping that it is the other party who needs help, and that all is well with his own world. In fact, the absentee one often plays the role of a victim of awful circumstances, accusing the other of being the game spoiler. It is very convenient to focus on the other because the more one does that, the less time one has to look at one's own warts and weak spots. It is a lazy way out because it does not take much effort to label the other as a flawed specimen of humanity.

My next meeting with Rani and Roopa, after a gap of a week, started with somewhat more ease and comfort than the first two had. This happens because initially the client is in a state of emotionality and rationality is missing. It is like being surrounded by thunder clouds, with the mind buffeted between one thought and another; the balance of mind is totally lost and feelings predominate. Once the client has vented hir/her feelings in two, three or sometimes more sessions, without being judged or directed, and only being heard and listened to with empathy and understanding, the degree of emotionality reduces and a bit of clarity begins to dawn.

In this meeting, another issue emerged. Ramesh had moved to the UK for higher studies. Under pressure from Roopa's father, he and Roopa had decided to call off their relationship, realizing the stakes were too high for them to handle. Meanwhile, Roopa, who had been applying for MBA courses in and out of the country, had been given a seat at a

All I want is a Fair Boy

business school in London. When she broke the news to her parents, however, hoping to receive congratulations on her achievement, her father vetoed the plan saying it would rekindle the passion between Roopa and Ramesh since both would be in the same country. Roopa pleaded with her father, saying they had given up their relationship and that they would be living in different cities.

There was no way her father was willing to buy any argument to allow her to go to the UK. Rani cried as she told me Roopa had decided to defy her father and declared that come what may, she was not going to miss out on the opportunity of studying in a good university. Things were indeed messy in their lives but it was too early for me as a counsellor to intervene. They needed to vent their emotions more. Nothing I said would make any sense at this early stage of counselling. The first few sessions give an opportunity for rapport building between strangers – the therapist and the client. It takes that long to vent and build confidence before clients feel secure enough to start opening the inner recesses of their hearts, layer by layer. It is not for the therapist to find solutions or direct the thinking of the client. When things do not go right, it is not the counsellor who is left holding the baby.

It is the therapist's job to provide insights to the client that he might have missed. It is the therapist's role not only to help the client make responsible choices but to also learn to face the consequences of those choices. The counsellor also attempts to convert those who are in victim roles (like Roopa and Rani), to learn to face the world on their own and turn from being victims to being victors. The counsellor's efforts are towards converting them from being doormats into persons of self worth. This is best done by giving them unconditional love, warmth and regard. Often, these are things they have not experienced. As consistent love and respect engulfs them, they begin to believe in themselves. A wise person once said this beautifully: "As a therapist, I am a companion. I try to help people tune into their own wisdom."

All I want is a Fair Boy

In the third session, I was hoping to see the father but he was too busy to come. There is always a temptation to take a judgmental position on absentee clients – the missing husband in the marital case, the father who is too busy to turn up for a meeting, or the adolescent boy who refuses to come for counselling but (according to his parents) stands in need of it. This is the time to take a deep breath and say to oneself, 'Hey, I am judging without even meeting the person, am I not?'

The third session with the mother and daughter was a repetition of what they had told me earlier. The week had gone past with the father becoming more belligerent and the daughter being equally stubborn. Roopa said that if her father would not support the idea of her going abroad, she would seek financial help from her sister and pay her back when she herself started earning. The mother was caught in a vice between the two. Her head was with her husband, the provider of the family, and her heart with her daughter. She was literally torn emotionally into pieces and did not know what to do.

We talked about the various options available to them and the consequences of those choices. Would the mother stand by the daughter? "Not possible," was the answer. Would the daughter change her mind and study in India? "Not possible," was the answer. Would the father change his position? "Not possible," was the answer. After discussing the choices and finding no light at the end of the tunnel, we decided to meet the coming week and I again conveyed my wish to see the father. As they were leaving, I gave them a ray of hope by saying that in such cases, my experience had taught me that resolution is usually possible.

Why weekly meetings and not more frequent ones? There are no fixed rules about this. The counsellor takes a call on the urgency and frequency. Obviously a suicidal case requires more frequent meetings than say, a case of anxiety. Also, a break of a week gives both the client and the counsellor time to reflect over the issues. Reflection, as mentioned earlier, is very important in this field.

In the fourth session, Roopa's father did come. He took centre stage by declaring he had been telling both women that what was going on at home was a family issue and had to be sorted out internally; that they were wasting my time and theirs by washing their dirty linen in public. "I am sure they have put all the blame on me. Look, Mr. Kumar, I have given this girl and her sister all the best things in life – education, cars, clothes, cell phones, and holidays. You name it and she has it. I have asked her for only one thing and she has reacted so rebelliously that I am shocked. All I have told this silly girl is to get married to a boy from our caste, who is an MBA, who is fair, and who is willing to look after my business when I cannot." He went on to explain that his first daughter had deserted them and moved to the U.S. Then he threw a direct question at me: "Do you think it is unfair of me to ask her for this much after all I have done for her?"

It took some time to explain to the father that the counsellor is neither an arbiter nor a judge. At best, he is a facilitator. We discussed various options such as the mother staying in London with the daughter for the initial months of Roopa's education, or frequent visits back home since money was not an issue. We talked about trusting his daughter since she had given her word that she had broken off with the boy, which she kept repeating in this session too. Roopa sobbed endlessly. The desperation on her face was heart rending. The mother looked down and I could see her tears dropping onto the floor. All I could do was to give them some tissues and water to help them deal with their trauma. The session ended with no conclusion being reached except to meet again the next week.

It crossed my mind that I was perhaps seeing a narcissistic person in the father. Readers may wonder that just a while ago an important point was being made about not judging the client, and here I am, in one session, labelling the client as a narcissist. Well, there are views and views on what judgment in counselling means. Being non-judgmental for me does not mean not having a fix on the kind of personality you are dealing with. However, this must be verified, checked and rechecked before a final position is taken. Judgment means not accepting the person for what he is. In some cases husbands and wives admit to having extra marital relationships, which is clearly adultery and against the law. Does that mean that we do not judge the person as an adulterer? What it means is that even though he has committed adultery, he is accepted as a person. He does not come down in my eyes as a human being. I might disagree about what he has done or is doing, but he is still a person of worth who needs help, consideration, love and regard. That is what makes the person regain his composure and self-worth.

Narcissism

Since I have mentioned that I could see some traces of narcissism in Roopa's father, this may be the time to explain a little about narcissism. Narcissists generally love themselves to the exclusion of all others. They consider themselves as a special gift to others and regard them as extensions of themselves. They are so totally absorbed in themselves that the feelings of others do not count. Narcissism, in its extreme form, has been described as malignant narcissism by Eric Fomm. It is very difficult to counsel narcissists because their love for themselves is greater than an alcoholic for his bottle. But like an alcoholic, he too can change when he hits rock bottom and says to himself, 'My God, what have I done to myself?' Similarly, narcissists change only when faced with extreme circumstances beyond their control, such as failure in business or marriage, or loss of face.

The father attended one more session and then called it quits. In the subsequent sessions with mother and daughter (the majority of them with the daughter alone), we discussed the choices and the consequences of each choice. Finally, after three sessions, Roopa decided she would give up her dream of going to the UK to study. The cost in terms of her father's pain, was too much for her to bear. She enrolled at a local college to do her MBA but remained in counselling to gain more confidence as a person and regain her lost self-esteem.

She was becoming more confident, positive and cheerful, and we were still working in that mode of counselling when she stopped coming for her sessions without any information.

In counselling, a percentage of counselees – statistically about 20% – stop coming when they realize that the change required is too great for them to handle and staying in the same known cocoon is more comfortable than changed circumstances. Take, for example, a case where the wife is physically and verbally abused and the only way after all options have been considered, is divorce, yet she prefers to stay in an abusive marriage rather than charter a new and unknown course in life. Such a person might stop coming for further sessions.

Counsellors, particularly less experienced ones, ought to remember that a client dropping out without notice is no reflection on their work, as long as they have done it with love, warmth and positive regard. There was a sad reason for Roopa dropping out, which I learnt later when she rang me after a month's absence to say her father had suffered a heart attack and passed away. Mother and daughter came back for counselling to cope with their grief.

COPING CAPACITY

'Cope' is an important word in counselling. Each person has a coping capacity, coping mechanism and coping skills, to deal with external pressures. Sometimes, due to various reasons, our coping mechanism and capacity is weaker than the external triggers we are faced with. Loss of a dear one, a job, loss of face, of a business, rejection by a loved one, and many other such triggers, can put a mentally healthy person into deep depression. Counselling helps, and in such cases where psychiatric intervention is required, a counsellor can be a bridge between the specialist and the client.

In most emotional problems, a little help is a lot of help.

All I want is a Fair Boy

Guruspeak: narcissism & difficult clients

In simple terms, narcissism can be described as self-absorption and being a prisoner of self-ego. Let me make one point clear: some traces of narcissism are present in all of us to maintain our self-esteem but when it becomes a personality disorder, it is time to worry. Narcissists react aggressively and with total denial, arrogance and conceit. They also show a tendency to envy others. Such people upset counsellors and therefore, the clan of counsellors should be aware of the negative transference taking place. You will have noticed in the case of Roopa's father, his tendency was to dictate 'my way or the highway', because narcissists have a sense of entitlement. They lack empathy and understanding towards others.

Remember Roopa's father asked: Is it too much to ask my daughter to marry a fair boy, from our community, who is ready to take over my business? Going by the book on the personality disorder issues, he would be considered a borderline narcissistic personality. This is how Widiger and Francis, famous mental health experts describe pathological narcissism: 'Behaviour characterised by expression of grandiosity, entitlement, exploitation, shallowness, low empathy, preoccupation with fame, wealth or grand achievements'. They add: '…they are conceited, arrogant but also envious of others including those who are satisfied with simple but meaningful lives.'

There are times a counsellor might not know enough about some personality disorder traits. It is best to consult someone who does, in order to understand better. I have a psychiatrist friend and often consult him when I fall short on knowledge or details.

Difficult Clients

Eugene Kennedy and Sara Charles, in their excellent book on counselling, *On becoming a counsellor*, have categorised some difficult-to-deal-with clients. Roopa's father was one such. In the context of counselling, such clients are termed *Reluctant Clients* and it is very important to enrol them into the process of counselling. Till the belief in the process itself is established, one cannot hope to see much traction in counselling. There is another category called *Resistant Clients*, who ask for help but not seriously. Their actions suggest they do not want couselling but come because they are led there by someone or because they get a lot of attention. They are comfortable with their drawbacks so long as they can continue to function in their lives. There are some who hide behind humour because they do not want to reveal much about their life's realities. Yet another category is *Talking Clients*, who talk about everything on earth but their real problems. They avoid saying anything about the real issues. But the category that can get a counsellor's goat is the *Intellectual Debater*. They will generalize, talk about the past and the future, and keep saying 'you know what I mean'. These clients need to be told firmly that we do not know what they mean. It is perfectly in the domain of a counsellor to withdraw himself and state clearly that there is not much he can do to help.

Attributes of a counsellor

Let us shift our focus from the client to the counsellor. It has been brought out that empathy and paraphrasing skills are important attributes of a counsellor. Here we will discuss a few other attributes a counsellor should possess to enhance his effectiveness. These are based on the findings of Robert Carkhuff, and I could not agree with them more, having found these attributes extremely useful in my own counselling career.

Genuineness & Immediacy

Genuineness in what we say and do must be reflected in our relationship with the client. Immediacy in our responses to the client's need is another factor. By immediacy, I mean that the counsellor's response should have spontaneity and potency. These attributes are essential for counsellors and can be learnt over time.

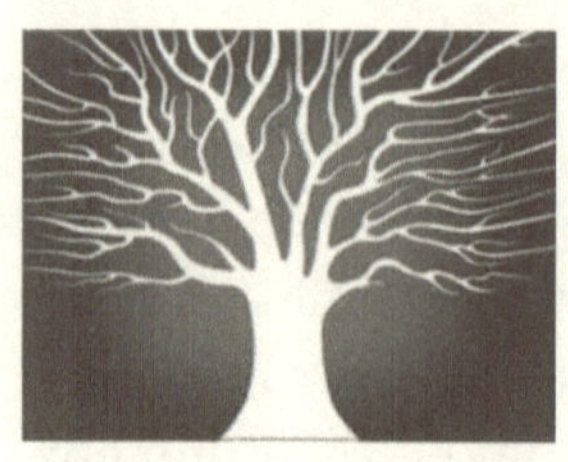

Now is the age of anxiety. ~ W H Auden

It was dusk when I saw two young boys walking up and down the pavement. I left them to their own devices. After waiting more than ten minutes, I got up to make inquiries about why they were there. Pointing to the other, the younger of the two told me that his brother needed help but was scared to get into counselling. I spontaneously asked the older boy whether I looked scary. His response was a feeble smile. I put an arm round his shoulders and escorted him into my counselling chamber. The younger brother made himself comfortable in a chair placed under a tree outside.

I introduced myself. This is one way of breaking the ice, and prompts clients to introduce themselves as well. Gopal was all of 22, well built and six feet tall, but his body language did not match his frame and his voice even less so. He was fidgety and his posture suggested he was uncomfortable talking about his issue to a total stranger. From the looks of him, he had not shaved for some days. Anxiety was written all over Gopal's face. For a counsellor, such clues are very important to observe. Body language gives a lot of information. It also points to contradictions sometimes, such as when the client displays low energy but says he is feeling fine. Counsellors, when appropriate, bring out this contradiction between body language and the spoken word. The technical term for this is 'confrontation'. The counsellor 'confronts' the client about the difference between what he sees and hears.

Gopal began his narrative: He had gone to Hubli to attend a wedding with his family and friends. They had a whale of a time and on the final day, after the wedding dinner, they were all enjoying themselves when one of them suggested someone should go and get *paans* (betel nuts

All it Needed was a Pinch of Tobacco

packed in green leaves). Each one placed their order, some wanting sweet, some *saada* (simple), and others asked for the tobacco-laden variety. Gopal asked for *meetha* (sweet). The paans were duly brought back and handed over. Gopal swallowed his *paan* and the next moment he was convulsing and having continuous hiccups. It was then his friends realized Gopal had been given a *paan* with tobacco.

As often happens with youngsters, Gopal became the butt of jokes for his friends, who called him a sissy because he could not eat a *paan* with a wee bit of tobacco. Gopal broke into a nervous sweat and truly believed he had suffered a heart attack because he felt pain in his chest and the convulsions would not stop. He excused himself, went to his room and tried to sleep, but could not because of the scary and persistent thought that if he went to sleep he would die. The next day, he travelled with the marriage party, by bus, back to Bangalore. All through the journey he was quiet and tormented with the incessant thought that he would die of heart attack at any moment. He did his best to push the thought from his mind but the more he tried, the more it persisted.

The only person he could share his pain with was his younger brother. He did not say a word to his parents in case they called him stupid or someone who worried over nothing. He was apprehensive about their response that it was foolish to think one little pinch of tobacco could cause a heart attack. Something we need to remind ourselves as often as we can, is that we have no right to challenge the reality of others. What is real to them may not appear real to us and vice versa. If we challenge the reality of another, then we give them permission to challenge our reality as well.

Counselling process: Attending phase

I want to break this narrative to share some thoughts on the counselling process. Counselling is a chaotic process. It has a beginning, middle and end, but if you think these happen in sequence, in properly segmented sections, in a linear way, then your assumptions are wrong. Even if you have moved from one stage of the process to another, it does not mean the client will not return to square one. That is why I use the word 'chaotic'. Having said that, there *is* a method to the chaotic pattern and it can be divided into various phases, as suggested by Robert R. Carkhuff in his book, *The Art of Helping in the 21st century.*

The first phase is sometimes called the *Attending Phase*. This phase helps to build rapport between the client and the counsellor. You attend to the client right from the time of his entry, through the initial narrative. Attending means leaning forward to hear the client with total attention while making eye contact that is friendly and non-threatening. Sitting squarely with a comfortable distance between counsellor and counselee, in an open and relaxed posture, also helps to attend.

Back to Gopal. He told me in the first and subsequent sessions, that his condition had gone from bad to worse. He would miss going to his recently-found job because he was scared he would die on the way, while riding his motor bike. The situation became so bad that one day, going to work, he felt he was having a heart attack. He got down, rested by the wayside, parked his bike there, and returned home in an auto rickshaw. There was also the problem of keeping his condition a secret from his parents. He had withdrawn to minimise his contact with them. Soon he began to limit his outings to a few hundred metres from home because he felt that if anything did happen to him, the chances were greater that he would be recognized by someone and be brought home safely. Dusk was like death to him. So he stopped stirring from home after dark. He felt safe confined to his room. He was mortally and perpetually scared of death. As time passed, the situation became even worse and more intense. Going out in the evening meant having his younger brother be his escort. That was the reason why, whenever he came to see me, his brother always accompanied him.

Readers may wonder and say to themselves, 'Hold on! One little episode can't be such a big thing. Gopal is a sissy and has become a shirker. Others have gone through greater hell, even near death experiences. In comparison, Gopal has gone through nothing. One proper dressing down would set him right.' To those entertaining such thoughts, I must say this: Don't be so sure my friend, that one day you will not be sitting in front of a counsellor with an issue smaller than what Gopal was facing. You cannot compare any two cases. I will go along with you if you can show me two human beings who are exactly the same. Each is atypical.

In life there are many external triggers (in this case, a tobacco-laden *paan*). How we cope with such triggers depends on our coping ability at that point of time. If the external trigger effect is stronger than our coping skill at that time, we are vulnerable and may need help. If it is the other way round and your coping skills are stronger than the trigger pressure, you will sail through. I would go so far as to say that, that is really the difference between client and counsellor. The counsellor is in better control of his life at this point of time, has better discriminating power, has energy, and is in a state of positivity. There are those who can take the pressures of life better than others. But the ability to cope with stress is not gifted to counsellors in any special way. They have to work hard at building their coping skills by living a balanced life of exercise, meditation, yoga, discussing their issues when they are in doubt, and having a social support network.

It was clear by now that Gopal had a streak of obsessive compulsive personality, which among other things, means that once a thought enters the mind, it is difficult to drive it out – particularly negative thoughts. For three sessions I heard him out, and as the third session ended, I knew the normal approach of providing insight would not work here. Gopal was not in an emotional state, he was clear and logical in what he was saying, except that he did not know how to drive away this obsessive, recurring thought from his mind.

Driving back home, I felt the typical counselling approach would not work for Gopal but self-disclosure might. I had gone through an almost identical experience three decades back. I made up my mind

All it Needed was a Pinch of Tobacco

to take the self-disclosure approach, in which the counsellor reveals something about himself to help the client. But a few caveats apply. The first and foremost is that the self-disclosure must be authentic and appropriate. It must also contribute to solidify the rapport between client and therapist. Also, self-disclosure must be discreet and never used for self-aggrandisement.

In the fourth session I told Gopal that it was strange but I had gone through a similar experience about three decades ago, and in some ways it had been more intense than his own experience. Of course, at the time I did not know anything about counselling or obsessive compulsive behaviour. I narrated my real life story: It was 1974 and I was 37 years old. I was in the Indian Air Force, healthy and fit. One afternoon, while having a nap, I had a terrible dream that I had had a heart attack. I got up with a start and started sweating. I was very nervous and told my wife I thought I had had a heart attack. She called her father, who lived not far from where we did, and in less than half an hour he walked in with a close friend of his, a doctor whom I had met on a few occasions. The doctor checked me out and declared me to be hale and hearty, and attributed my worry to a bad dream. Having made his diagnosis, he had a hearty laugh and left, with the final advice that I have a brandy before going to sleep. I would get up feeling better. I must say that I was relieved, but only through that evening.

The thought that my heart attack was real and not a figment of my imagination, persisted with me and I could not share it with anyone. I could not tell my wife because I was always seen as a macho Air Force guy. How could I admit to falling prey to such weak thinking? I was the problem-solver of the family. How could I admit my own helplessness? I could not confide in the Air Force doctor lest I be hospitalised and downgraded medically. I suffered in silence. I started taking medicines to calm my nerves and finally summoned up the courage to tell my wife. I started seeing civilian doctors on the sly and went through an ECG and treadmill test, which showed a healthy heart. That assurance lasted in my mind for a forthright, and then I had a panic attack and underwent another check, this time a lumbar puncture. I was even hypnotised to get to the bottom of my problem. But all these procedures gave me a clean chit. But the mind can be a bigger devil than we imagine. Once it decides to torment us, it does not let go. One cannot show it the treadmill, or the ECG declaring you as fit as an athlete, and hope it will buy the argument.

I would find my index finger rubbing my chest in the heart area, so much so that my shirts became faded and frayed there. It came to the stage when I could produce the signs of a heart attack at will. I came close to committing suicide more than once but did not have the courage to go ahead. Yes, suicide requires courage and energy to execute. It is a myth that suicide is the act of someone weak and low on energy.

I narrated my war with my heart and mind to Gopal, who listened with rapt attention. He kept saying, "Really Uncle, this happened to you!" I had taken an authentic self-disclosure approach in this case. Gopal must have thought, 'If Sir went through this and came out a winner, and is a counsellor today, I too can win this battle'. But in my self-disclosure, I intentionally omitted to mention that it took me more than five years to deal with the issue, lest I discourage him. The counsellor's aim is to move the client from a state of hopelessness to one of hopefulness; from 'there is no alternative' to 'there is always an alternative', from TINA to TIAAA. Gopal asked me how I eventually solved the issue and I told him (in TV show style), that the next part of my story would be related after the break. We shook hands warmly like partners in crime, and parted. I could not help but notice a subtle change for the better.

I did not know I was using a behaviourist approach when I did what I did to deal with my long-festering issue. Running was my passion, as it is even today. I would be out every day, logging 10 kilometres. While running, I would tell my heart that if I was going to die because

All it Needed was a Pinch of Tobacco

of it, I would rather die on a running track than lying in bed. I would run faster to challenge my sick mind. One month followed another and I was still alive. Gradually, the overwhelming, ever-present and all-controlling thought began to lose its intensity. Mark the word 'gradually', because it took years to overcome my emotional trauma. There is always a rosy side (the other side of the coin), to all sorrows and mine was that this perpetual race with my heart turned me into a marathon runner.

I used the behaviourist approach to resolve my own issue. But there are many approaches in counselling. You cannot use a one-shoe-fits-all style, and even with the same client, the therapist calibrates the approach needed at a particular stage of counselling. Generally, my approach is to provide an insight that the client, in a state of emotionality, may have missed. He gets a new idea, acts on it, and watches whether it works for him. In the behaviourist approach, you do something, see it work, and become convinced in your mind. This is a very simple explanation of the approach.

To empathise with Gopal was not difficult for me. Empathy means getting under the skin of the person and into his shoes. I had once worn those shoes myself. When Gopal arrived for the next session, I did what I had not done before. I put on my walking shoes and invited him to walk with me. We talked about everything but the issue he was dealing with. I enrolled his brother for this task as well, on a daily basis, and told him not to rush the process but increase the nightly outings at the level Gopal was comfortable with. I continued seeing him every week, more to keep his case under review.

Then one day, Gopal asked his brother to come into the chamber. The young boy walked in with a box of sweets. Gopal said that he felt confident enough to manage his life now. I gave him a hug, saw him to the gate, and told him that if he ever needed my help, I was always there for him. This is a necessary assurance a client needs to receive at the time of parting. Often, they do need help again. Walking back to my chamber I once again thought I was truly blessed that life was running well for me. This is a thought almost all counsellors admit to after the day's sessions.

Talking of counsellors, depending on the intensity of the case, a counsellor can become stressed and overwhelmed by the end of a session or after a few sessions. This happens more often to relatively new counsellors. When this occurs, counsellors are advised to vent their feeling to their co-counsellors.

COUNSELLING PROCESS: RESPONDING STAGE

I have mentioned various stages of counselling and that the first is the *attending stage*. The next is the *responding stage*. Each stage requires different skill sets, such as getting information out of the client, observation, and many others. However, common to all – and the most important among them – is listening. This listening is active and has no filter and jammers; it expresses interest and empathy; is total and without distraction, such as looking at the door or the/a watch.

The vital listening skill in the responding stage is the ability to paraphrase what the client is saying, so the person gets the message: Yes, he can see my world. Yes, he can see where I am coming from. Yes, he has captured my feelings exactly. It is unlikely that a person who cannot experience his own feelings will be able to pick up those of another. If you have not burnt your fingers over a flame, it is unlikely that you will understand the pain caused by a burn. If you have not felt guilt or helplessness, you will find it difficult to capture exactly those feelings in another.

Also essential, is the skill of observing appearance and behaviour. In addition, the skill of concentrating on the feeling, by responding appropriately, is very important: 'You feel angry your parents don't give you the same consideration they give to your brother.' Or 'You feel sad that despite your best efforts, your mother-in-law does not appreciate you.' The responses should be simple.

All it Needed was a Pinch of Tobacco

A BIT ABOUT THE OBSESSIVE STYLE

In Gopal's case, I used the term called 'obsessive compulsive'. This may be a good time to dig deeper into this trait. All of us have a bit of it but it does not impede our day-to-day life. Obsessive are recurring thoughts like Gopal had, which cannot be driven away either by force or voluntarily. And compulsion is a habit or impulse you cannot resist – like washing your hands over and over again, cleaning up the kitchen not once, not twice, but many times. It is something you may not want to do but still do because you are obsessed. Compulsion is something that you check and recheck repeatedly. Some people check their manuscript repeatedly until the writing becomes lifeless, soulless and mechanical.

Anxiety is an integral part of the obsessive compulsive personality. Such people are rigid, formal, and often stiff. They feel guilty about enjoying life. They can argue their case and intellectualise every situation. Offence is the best defence in their strategy. They tend to sulk and be quiet to get even with others. In short, they are not easy to counsel. Therefore, the behaviour modification approach works best with them, as in Gopal's case. Stir out for a short distance, increase the distances on an incremental basis, feel comfortable, and move further. You can call it the fake-it-till-you-make-it approach.

GURUSPEAK: OBSESSIVE COMPULSIVES & ANXIETY OBSESSION

In extreme cases, the following signs manifest themselves. There is rigidity in the pattern of living and the clients are dogmatic and opinionated in their thinking. They are stiff and formal and lack the ability to relax and enjoy life even though they may have the means to do so. Obsessive compulsives try to get on top of each situation and are unhappy with half measures. They practice and practice before making a public appearance, like giving a speech. Security in life is more important to them than satisfaction. It is hard to connect with them at the emotional level because they tend to intellectualize situations. It is useless to try and win arguments with them. Counsellors find it difficult to connect with them at the feelings-level because they insulate themselves. They even ask counsellors to explain why they said what they did.

In extreme cases, they get obsessive thoughts about something that they do not want to do, like hurting someone. But the idea horrifies them and they do not execute their thoughts. But that is not to say the same thoughts do not invade them at intervals. Once again, in extreme cases, they go about rechecking the things they have done, arranging and rearranging their work stations. They are not easily satisfied and want to do better and better. They are aware of their compulsive habits/acts but cannot do much about them. Also, their behaviour leads to neurosis. You will see them trying to constantly maintain control over themselves. Loss of control means failure to them. They are comfortable only when they feel they know everything about a subject. Offence is the best form of defence for obsessive compulsives. Do not be surprised if you get a tutorial from them on how to improve your counselling knowledge and skills. Beware of the irritation that counselling such persons can cause you. Do not let them hijack your happiness or control in the counselling sessions. In short, obsessive compulsives are a great challenge for counsellors.

A FEW FACTS ABOUT ANXIETY

Lay counsellors are not expected to delve deep into the psychological adaptation of their clients. That is usually left to specialists like clinical psychologists or psychiatrists. But my personal experience tells me that it helps to establish a psychological fix on the client, otherwise the counsellor might apply a one-size-fits-all approach. For example, I would not apply the same counselling approach to a narcissist as I would to an obsessive compulsive personality.

If you know the psychological domain of the client, you also know the reason behind their responses. The narcissist might come across as someone who thinks the whole universe revolves around him. An obsessive compulsive might stay grooved in the same position. That is not to say one can always be sure of the frame of reference of the client. Even experts in the field agree on that.

All it Needed was a Pinch of Tobacco

In the case of Gopal, I mentioned that he was behaving like an obsessive compulsive personality. On the other hand, he could have been a case of high level anxiety. This era has been named 'the age of anxiety'. To be anxious while crossing a road or flying through turbulent weather is understandable, but when our responses are disproportionate to the happenings around us, then it becomes neurotic anxiety. Healthy fear is one thing, but to be fearful in all situations is something else.

The one thing that counsellors ought to remember is that one cannot ask the client to wish away their anxiety. They feel vulnerable. In one case the person may be anxious but soon deals with it, while in another case, he may experience runaway anxiety, with the heartbeat and pulse rate soaring. Gopal's behaviour could well relate to anxiety. The idea is not to push such clients too far or too early. One should not be too demanding of them. Allow them to set their own pace. If we find a person's reaction to a situation is totally out of proportion, it could be a case of neurotic anxiety. Their reality is different. For them, anxiety is real and cannot be wished away.

You will have met people who do everything to avoid the surgeon's knife, even though it is the recommended option to resolve their medical problem. Anxiety can play havoc on the mind. More and more people are resorting to popping pills to manage their anxiety, but the long-term side effects can take a toll and create adverse effects and dependency.

A client's anxiety attacks can stress counsellors as well, because often the person suffering from anxiety cannot even pinpoint the reason for his anxiety. There is a tendency to advise the anxious to drive out their fears. But better results are obtained through understanding the person and letting him vent his fears. Over time, anxiety dissolves with understanding and encouragement from the counsellor.

Listening is when we give up our thoughts and interests for a while to be able to give full attention to the other. ~ Anonymous

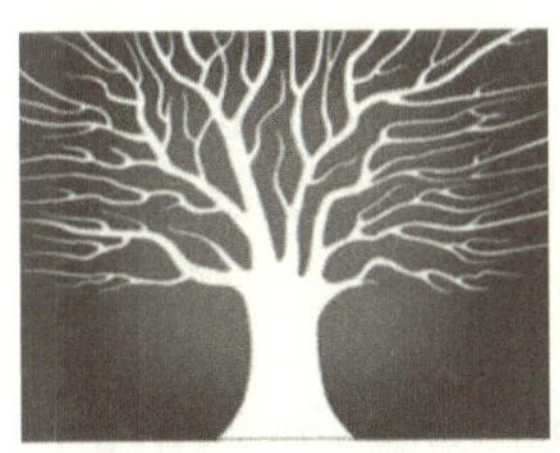

Sensual pleasures have the fleeting brilliance of a comet; a happy marriage has the tranquillity of a lovely sunset. ~ Ann Landers

The next case lasted just seven sessions, and the client stopped consultation abruptly without giving me any indication why. I have mentioned the contribution of Freud and his pioneering role in psychotherapy. Over time, as in all disciplines and philosophies, many other approaches to counselling/therapies have emerged over the years. These include Transactional Analysis, Reality Therapy, Behavioural Conditioning, Rational Emotive and Gestalt. Some are complimentary to each other while others take different approaches. But each works in its own way. Sometimes experienced counsellors mix and match these disciplines, depending on the need of the client at that point in time. We will not go into the details of these different counselling philosophies here but as we delve deeper into counselling approaches, we will study the various options that can be brought to the table to help a client.

The fact remains that the world over, about 80% of transient mental disturbances are taken care of by lay counsellors. We are not talking here of deeply disturbed people who are neurotic (sometimes described as people who wish that they were Mahatma Gandhi), or psychotic (those who claim to be Mahatma Gandhi). An expert once described neurotics as those who build castles in the air and psychotics as those who move around in them. And psychiatrists collect the rent. We are also not talking about clients with mental illness, like the deeply depressed, hallucinating or schizophrenic; or those with personality disorders, like obsessives, histrionics, paranoids or narcissists. For want of a simpler description, I have put them in the 'mental fracture' category. These people need specialised help from a qualified psychiatrist, along with medication. However, lay counsellors can certainly give relief to these professionals by taking on 'mental sprains' like stress, anxiety, marital discord, adolescence, mild depression and interpersonal relationship issues.

It is well established that about 80% of clients gain from the help they receive from counsellors. The remaining 20%, clients find it difficult to move from their current positions to projected positions. The pain of change is more than the pain of remaining the same. It could also be that the counsellor is ineffective. Such a counsellor is not happy with his own life, has been a mere observer, or concentrates more on the problem than on the person before him. A counsellor must never forget that behind every problem there is a human being. The client has the right to choose the counsellor and should indeed terminate sessions if he does not have sufficient trust and confidence in that particular counsellor.

Attributes of a counsellor

There are certain attributes a counsellor is expected to possess. Some essential qualities are: empathy, compassion, understanding, acceptance of others, positive regard for others, and a state of congruence with themselves, in that they are well rounded (not physically!), well grounded, and comfortable with themselves. They should be happy to help. However, if there is one quality a counsellor *must* possess, that clearly is the ability to actively listen.

Besides ensuring confidentiality and a non-judgmental approach, counsellors do not usually direct their clients to take steps in one direction or the other. As the consequences of doing so are borne by the client, it is the client who needs to decide which direction his life should take. The counsellor's task is to help him take the decision. For example, say I as a counsellor was to advise a married woman who had tried all other options, to go in for a divorce, and she does so only to find her post-divorce life even worse than her married life was, with all its ups and downs and upheavals, who would manage

From One Bed to Another

her affairs? Insight, yes. Advice, no. Guidance, yes. Discussing options and even throwing up options, yes. But decisions, no. Take another example: A young boy has problems that can easily be traced to a deficiency in parenting. His parents can be guided or enrolled to undergo therapy, but if they decline, it is their choice and so are the consequences of the choice.

Now, coming to the case under discussion, it was a young and pretty girl in her early twenties who walked into my office with confidence and asked if I was free to see her. As I responded in the affirmative, one look told me the young woman was either an actress or a model, and I had a vague impression that I had seen her somewhere. There were two other indicators that she was different from the people who generally come to me for counselling. Unlike most others, she was confident, and dressed for an evening engagement, after meeting me. She came straight to the point, saying that she frequently got trapped by young boys who professed love and thrust attentions upon her. However, after having full-blown affairs, they would suddenly disappear. These were the pre-cell phone days where tracing a truant lover was thrice as difficult as it is today.

In the next three sessions she told me of her experiences. Abridged, the narration flowed something like this: A young boy from Haryana ('these young men from the North', was a phrase she commonly used), chatted her up one evening in a social setting. She volunteered to tell him something about her life, work, work place, and working hours. Then one evening, the young man was waiting for her at the office gate, sitting on his motorbike. He suggested they go out for a a spin and perhaps spend the evening together. She said she had some doubts about going ahead, but without giving the proposal much thought, sat on the pillion and they drove off to a restaurant and had a few snacks. Over time, it became common practice for her to be, literally, taken for a ride, from her office to bed in a three-bedroom flat the boy shared with a number of college mates. It was fun living this could-not-care-less life. I should mention that in her spare time, she modelled for a jewellery shop and her picture perfect poster was on display in the centre of town. She did not say so but it was apparent she was quite enjoying her life.

The subsequent part of her life's play went like this: One day, the young man broke contact without giving reason or notice. He just disappeared. She took the runaway episode in her stride and continued her life as if nothing had happened. Yes, she was angry. Yes, she felt she had been used. Yes, she had been fooled. But she felt these things happened sometimes. She was direct in her question when she asked me: "It happens sometimes, doesn't it?" Even with all my experience and skills in impromptu communication, I was stumped and said that frankly I had no experience in this regard.

Then, one not-so-fine evening, she found another young man waiting for her outside the gate of the office on his bike. He told her that his dear friend from Karnal, her first beau, had asked him to deliver a message to her. She decided to have a cup of coffee with this total stranger. She was very keen, she said, to know about the mystery of the disappearance of her first beau. The mystery remained unsolved but a new contact was established. The messenger became her new lover. And it did not stop at that. Some of the rich boys in the group began inviting her to fancy hotels in the city for late night binges. They had money to splurge and she enjoyed the attention and five star luxuries, which as a secretary in a medium-sized company, were beyond her reach. The young boys wanted a decent return on their investment and she had only her body to give.

She was hurt by the way she was being treated as a commodity but there was nothing in her behaviour to put an end to this round robin from one bed to another. When I asked her why she was allowing herself to be used in this manner, her defence was that if she did not agree, the boys were capable of blackmailing her. So she continued, until one evening she was in for a big surprise. She went to the flat to seek some clarification from one of the boys she had bedded. She was stopped at the door by a woman who said that the boy was with one of her girls and that she was not to go inside. She roamed the corridor until the coast was clear and then charged into the room and expressed her anger at his behaviour. The boy explained that he was feeling very lonely, being so far from home, and he fell into the temptation of engaging a prostitute. What she said next was the shocker. The same evening, she herself bedded the boy and had full-blown sex with him.

Is the thought going through your mind that all this cannot be true? How could an educated girl fall into one trap after another? If you are thinking on those lines, stop, because each of us is unique and different. We cannot apply our yardstick to another. In my mind, I was unclear how to move forward with the case. Sometimes I found myself doing and saying things that would improve her self-esteem. I would try and glide in the insight that she should try and see herself as a person of worth, a gift, someone special, instead of reducing herself to a mere object to be passed on for sexual gratification from one boy to another. I missed no chance to build her self-esteem by acknowledging everything she did right, from coming on time to reading some of the material I gave her on the subject. It made some difference but the main plot did not change

I began to suspect that there was a certain compulsiveness about her sexual behaviour and suggested she meet a sexologist and see what a person from that discipline had to say. She said she would go but then she stopped coming. I took it in my stride. It sometimes happens that the client, without giving any reason, stops showing up and does not even inform the counsellor. Novice counsellors sometimes take this as their personal failure. But with experience, they change their attitude to: 'I have given what I had to offer. I did my best. I am satisfied. I cannot chase the client to come back. That is not my job. They came of their own volition and it is their fundamental right to end counselling at the time of their choosing.'

The story of the young girl did not end there. Yes, she turned up one evening, this time looking very distraught. She said she had resigned from her job and gone into hiding for some months to escape the "North Indian gang", as she put. Later, on the recommendation of a family friend, she had become the personal secretary of a political bigwig. She had not realized that the 'personal' part of her job would be taken seriously by her boss. The job called for her to travel with him to Delhi on his frequent jaunts – not to keep notes of his discussions with his political counterparts, but to wait for him in the hotel room to relieve the boss of the stresses he had gone through during the day. The compensation was living in luxury hotels and sleeping in four-poster beds with her boss. Things got worse when on these outstation trips, some friends of the boss also wanted their share of fun. She became fed up and came back to me for consultation. After two sessions, I did what came to my mind, and that was to move her to what in counselling is commonly known as the 'personalisation phase'.

PERSONALIZATION PHASE

Let me explain what 'personalisation' means. After the attending phase and the responding phase have been gone through, the client usually moves from an emotional phase to a rational phase. That is, the client begins to see his position or situation more clearly, and you find them using expressions like, 'I should be doing this', rather than, 'This was no way for my husband to behave'.

Instead of saying, 'She (the mother-in-law) is tormenting me', the client begins to think in terms of, 'What do I do now to deal with my mother-in-law? I realize that I can do nothing to her but I can do something to change my responses to her. I am going to take charge of my life. I shall not be a doormat that my mother-in-law can walk all over'. When the counsellor observes the client personalising the issue, and is willing to stop looking at herself as a victim of circumstances, or (to use a sporting term), the client decides to pick up the ball and play the game, the process of goal-setting is initiated. This involves deciding what the client will do, when he will do it, with whom, and by when the goal will be achieved. At the end of the day, the client has to admit that any other option is hell. He cannot spend all his life trying to modify the behaviour of others. The insight that the client receives is that even assuming one is successful in changing the behaviour of others, there is no guarantee that yet another person will not turn up to cause havoc in one's life.

I moved the model client to the personalising phase by asking her a simple question: What *she* was doing, or not doing, to find herself in the same, recurring, messy problem. She began protesting, saying that everyone was out to take advantage of her. I reminded her that when she found the boy was already having fun with a prostitute, nothing had stopped her from retracing her steps and coming back home, rather than choosing to wait for her turn and going into the room. She protested that instead of helping her, I was criticising her. I told her firmly that she had either to change her own behaviour or stop complaining. "You can't have both options – to keep entering bedrooms, and also keep complaining. Choose one. Change the behaviour or stop complaining." Awkward silence followed and the session ended. The girl stopped coming. This happens when the client is willing to live with the pain of the current life because the energy required to change is too great to summon. Like some wives who, even after counselling, continue to choose to live in abusive marriages rather than seek options like divorce.

Guruspeak: sexual   overdrive
I mentioned that in this case I had recommended the client visit a sexologist to get to the bottom of her situation. There are times when a counsellor needs to seek help from qualified professionals, in complicated cases where his own domain knowledge does not extend. Therefore, it helps to keep a referral list of qualified professionals to recommend in such cases.

There are one or two other points that need to be highlighted here. Although a lot of material is available on sexual inhibitions, the research on the subject of sexual overdrive seems rather limited. Could it be that while we view lower levels of desire as abnormal, we prefer to dismiss an over-active sexual life as a non-issue? Some believe that it has something to do with our genes, while other research says it may have something do with mental illness. There are some specialists who tell me that in the liberal environment that we live in, sexual overreach is beginning to be seen as an adventure. Others ask this question: Who decides how much is beyond the limit? There is also some loud thinking going on to the effect that an excess of sexual desire could be related to hormone imbalance.

But there is more and more convergence in the belief that sexual overdrive is an addiction people develop as they taste it. It can lead to a disastrous life. Just as an alcoholic gets a kick out of sipping a drink, people addicted to libido get a kick out of frequent sex. And the only way to deal with it is through counselling by cognitive theory, which means helping to change the thinking of the person; or by avoiding those situations which lead one to fall into a trap.

Counselling is readiness to empty ourselves of our own concerns in order to make room for those of others.

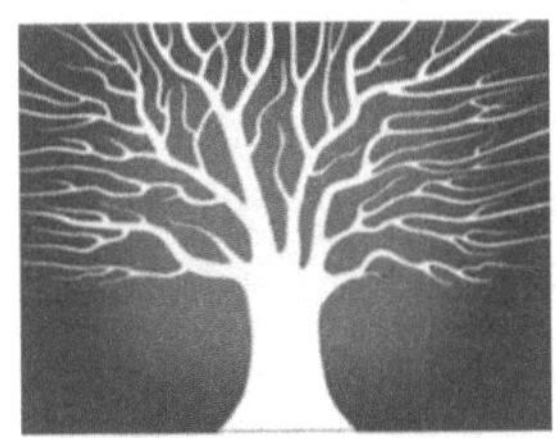

PUT SOME SENSE INTO THIS BOY'S HEAD

Just like other illnesses, depression can be treated, so that people can live happy, active lives. ~ Tom Bosley

This was the command I received from a father who had brought his son for counselling. He went on to explain that his son, in his early 30s, had become so lazy and disinterested that he had even started missing work, when he had once been regular. Over time, he had become aloof – so much so that he had moved from his bedroom to a small room located on the roof. There he lay, and had to be called down to get ready for work, eat breakfast, and leave for office. On many days, he would return in a couple of hours, climb up to the room, and lie staring at the roof. His personal hygiene had gone for a toss and he would neither shave nor bathe.

The father said he should have been stricter with his son when he first saw the signs of his turning into a work shirker and selfish man. He went on to say, "At the drop of a hat he gets angry with his mother, when the poor thing tries to do everything for him, like cooking the food he likes and taking care of his other needs. Put some sense into his head, and make sure he behaves appropriately for his age." I asked him what his own profession was and he said he was a retired Air Force officer. Suddenly his clear, commanding and authoritative tone began to make sense.

There are certain recommended ways to ask questions in counselling sessions. To probe in order to satisfy one's curiosity, is simply not done. Nor does one ask closed-ended questions, the answer to which is either 'no' or 'yes', as in the question: 'Was your father there at that time?' The answer, whether 'yes' or 'no', does not lead to understanding or enable

Put some Sense into this Boy's Head

exploration of the client's feelings. The best way to ask a question in counselling is to do it indirectly or by paraphrasing. For example: 'If I understand you right, you are very angry that you did not get the kind of support that you expected from your father'. The person might reply: 'Not exactly angry, but I was certainly very disappointed that my father did not come to help' or, 'Not only angry, but frustrated at the way my father behaved'. In this way, the counsellor can get in touch with the intensity and range of the feelings the client is going through.

Paraphrasing is a very important skill that needs more explanation. Assume that a young woman has come for counselling because her mother has decided to divorce her father and is preparing to move out. She says:

Client: I am very upset with my mother for wanting to divorce my father.

Counsellor: You are angry and upset over their separation.

Client: Yes, I don't know what has got into her head. Why would she want to leave my father?

Counsellor: You feel let down and your mother's decision makes no sense to you.

Client: Exactly. Particularly when my father is such a nice man and has done so much for us.

Counsellor: You feel your father has done nothing to deserve such an unfair decision.

Client: Exactly. I am confused what my future will be after this.

Counsellor: What pains you is that your mother's decision has made your future uncertain.

Readers will observe a few things here. First, the counsellor is capturing the thoughts and the feelings of the young woman and conveying them back to her. This is very important for two reasons: first, the client knows she is being understood and therefore it helps her to continue the narrative. It helps her vent her anger and the venting helps her regain her composure. The second point to be noticed is the words chosen by the counsellor are 'feeling' words like angry, upset, let down, confused, and pain. The idea is to capture the feelings and the intensity of those feelings. This helps to build rapport between the counsellor and counselee. No probing is being done here to satisfy the curiosity of the counsellor.

After meeting the father, I called the client into my chamber. I saw a young man with drooping shoulders, eyes fixed to the ground, unshaven and unkempt. The first thought that came to me was that I was perhaps looking at a depressed person. After greeting him, I asked Ravi what had brought him to me and if he could briefly tell me how life had been running for him. He said that his father had asked him to come. Full stop. No more conversation, just silence and looking down. As a counsellor, one knows it is best not to rush in to fill a gap or the silence of a client. Patience is required. Ravi's response to my next question, about the reason his father had brought him to me, was a deep sigh. A little later, he volunteered to tell me in a feeble voice that he had lost interest in life and his work. I paraphrased this and said, "You find not much purpose in life and it seems to drag on you". He responded by nodding.

Through the process of empathic listening and exploring his life over many sessions, this is what came out: Ravi worked in a manufacturing company. He was doing well in the purchase department. His boss was happy with him and would hold him up as a role model to the others. He was honest, a good negotiator, respectful with colleagues and suppliers. He called himself a self-starter who needed no goading and prodding to accomplish his tasks in time and well. The boss delegated a lot of work to him and Ravi got accelerated promotions. Life was hunky dory for Ravi, both at work and at home. In fact, he was beginning to think in terms of getting married, when one incident derailed him – and that was a change of boss.

His old boss moved up the corporate ladder and in his place came a replacement from another company. The DNA of the new boss was very different. He believed in shouting at people to get things done, blamed others in the presence of the whole group, took credit for things that had gone right, and trashed his subordinates when things went wrong. Everyone was fed up with him. He never had anything worthwhile to say to his colleagues (the term the previous chief had used; this one called them subordinates). He would tell them they would have to pay a heavy price for insubordination.

For Ravi, it was a big setback. He was compelled to go to the new boss to get approvals for everything, from buying small value hardware to high value steel. The boss would doubt his integrity, and sign the papers and fling them across the table. Unlike earlier, when he would sit across the table, the first time Ravi pulled the chair out to sit down, the new boss asked rudely whether he had been given permission to do so. "Don't take things for granted, understand?" the man shouted. This sudden change of environment was too much for Ravi, an upright and honest man, to bear. He started missing work and within a few days went into depression. All this came out over many sessions as his narrative was not coherent, logical or sequential.

The change of boss was the trigger that literally did Ravi in and he went deeper and deeper into depression. He had no interest in food, exercise, dress, socialising, or for that matter, in life. His desperation, he said in a very subdued voice, was such that he hated to see the sun rise, not knowing how to get through the day. I asked him if he saw no light at the end of the tunnel. His answer was that he saw no reason to live. To a direct question about whether he wanted to end his life, the response was an emphatic 'yes'.

It is not that all depressed people feel this way, but approximately 30% do consider and commit suicide. In Ravi's case, the trigger was the change of boss. He could not cope with it, while some others could. Here our concern is for those who come to us, because, as has been mentioned before, no two humans are the same. Also, the bandwidth of depression is different. It can range from an episode of sadness to deep psychotic depression requiring urgent medical help.

Put some Sense into this Boy's Head

Many other triggers happen in our lives which force us to enter the deep, dark hole of depression. For instance:

- Loss of confidence
- Death of a dear one
- Loss of face
- Loss of business
- Separation
- Helplessness due to age-related infirmities/protracted illness
- Something the person just cannot handle/adjust to, even promotion ('My God, will I be able to live up to the expectations of others?')

There are genetic and biological reasons for depression but those are best left to the medical professionals to discuss. My fond hope is that some day, an expert will write about mental illness issues in India and do so in language that high school students can understand.

It was soon clear to me that Ravi needed counselling, but more than that, he needed the intervention of a psychiatrist. The family resisted and had to be persuaded that it was for the wellbeing of Ravi that he be seen by a specialist. The reason for resistance is common in such cases. Any mention of a psychiatrist is taken as a sign of the person having traces of madness. It needs to be drilled into the family and close friends (we call them 'caregivers'), that they are doing harm to their dear ones in not seeking the help of a doctor, whose support is necessary in cases of deep depression. The counselling process must run parallel to the medication route.

The other thing caregivers need to be aware of is that it is extremely stressful to live with a depressed person. Moreover, since they are not aware of the subject, caregivers often do things – out of concern but also from ignorance – that harm rather than help the person. Caregivers too, need counselling to deal with the stress they undergo when dealing with the depressed.

Put some Sense into this Boy's Head

There are a few other things worth mentioning. The most important is for the caregivers to see that the medicines are administered to the patient as prescribed, and be aware that frequent consultations with the doctor are necessary. It is my experience that many times the caregivers take the patient off the medicines when they see progress, fearing that the person will get addicted to them. What they don't realise is that the patient will go back to square one and the whole process will have to be restarted. The thing to remember is that it is the doctor who prescribes medication and s/he is the only competent professional to take the patient off it. The insight that we need to give the caregivers is this: Which of the two is a better option? Taking medicine or living a depressed life? We also need to clarify that medicines are not addictive, as most of us tend to believe.

The last thing to do is to sermonize and say: 'Others have gone through much more difficult issues in their lives and handled them, and you are stuck with one episode. How long will this carry on like this?' The depressed person is burning inside and thinking: 'Who the hell cares about others, damn it. I am talking about me!' To challenge the reality of another is the most foolish thing one can do. Instead, we need to get into the shoes of that person and say: 'I were that person and gone through the same experiences, and if I was in a similar situation, my God, I wouldn't be any different.' Now that is empathy described in simple words.

Caregivers often tell us that the person in their care gets angry for no rhyme or reason, even when they are doing their very best. They need to know that anger is an integral part of the depressed. Such people have forgotten all the happy days of their life. For them, happiness never existed. We also need to make the caregivers aware of the fact that progress in the case of the depressed, is generally slow. 'Do not expect any gratitude in return,' is the message.

Coming back to the case of Ravi, he was referred to a doctor who, as expected, declared that he was indeed going through depression. But one complaint the parents made to me was that the doctor did not spend much time on the case and seemed to be in a hurry to dispense medicines. In the early phases of my practice, when I received such feedback about doctors, I would be livid and say to whoever cared to listen that that was no way to behave. But soon I discovered the following facts: the ratio of psychiatrists to patients is woefully low. The same is the case with the psychiatric bed-to-patient ratio.

One day, while talking to a doctor, I raised the issue. "I have to make a choice," he replied, "either spend more time with patients or cure more patients." It made sense. Therefore, counsellors need to do the counselling part, and if necessary, keep giving inputs to the doctor on their observations in the counselling room; while the doctor does his own bit. It becomes a joint venture in healing.

This was one of the longest cases that I have handled. Ravi and I met for thirty weekly sessions before he could be weaned off. In these sessions, it was my job to be in touch with his current reality and deal with the issues of the day. One of the insights that worked well was: just as the happy days of working with the gentle boss were not permanent, in the same manner the unhappy days of working with a difficult boss would also not be permanent. I worked on his self-esteem, talking about the good things he had achieved.

This case had a happy ending and it felt good to be invited to Ravi's wedding. Speaking of weddings, there is a common belief that marriage is a panacea for depressed people: *Shaadi kara doh toh sab theek ho jayega.* (Get him married and all will be fine.) No way! We keep reminding parents that marriage means only one thing – that instead of one family suffering, there will be two.

I used the word 'insight' because I believe that one of the main roles of a counsellor is to provide insights gently to the client – insights he may have missed. A few other points about the depressed:

- There is a loss of confidence and they have low energy, but want to get back to a healthy state quickly.

Put some Sense into this Boy's Head

- They have hostile feelings about the people around them.
- They get into self-punishment mode and it is very demanding working with them.
- They get angry seeing other people happy and any attempt to jolly them has exactly the opposite effect.
- They develop a co-dependency on the counsellor.
- Since they have time hanging on their hands and want to know what is going on with them, they read up a lot. They Google sites on depression, and often challenge and irritate the counsellor.

Whatever the responses of the client may be, it is the counsellor's aim to plant the seed of hope in the mind, both psychologically and medically.

There is something called manic or bipolar depression, the signs of which are: being on a high during one phase (full of energy; not in touch with reality; going on a buying spree much beyond one's financial limits; gifting presents by the dozens), and then plummeting downwards in the next phase. The second phase is marked by low energy, isolation, lack of interest, anger and emotional constriction. According to statistics, about fifteen percent of manic depressives end their lives by committing suicide.

There is a strong possibility of transference taking place in counselling the depressed. And also of counter-transference in the counsellor, who begins to find the client's behaviour irritating. False heartiness and jollying up the depressed person can be harmful. While counselling, the counsellor has to take an active role. The process is very slow, and empathic ties between the counsellor and the depressed client have to be strong. However, experienced counsellors are also aware that however slow the progress may seem, it *is* taking place.

GURUSPEAK: DEPRESSION

Experts in the domain of mental health remind us that dealing with the depressed is also depressing. Moving forward from the current

Put some Sense into this Boy's Head

position to a desired position, something a counsellor desires from the client, requires internal energy. And that is something that is depleted in a depressed person. A friend of mine in Delhi would have long conversations with me on every subject on earth, including politics, business, movies, children, while driving to work. He would put on loud music in his car and ask me to listen to a song that he knew was my favourite. He was never in a hurry to end the conversation until I stopped him. Then came depression. With it came only monosyllablic replies. This is the kind of change a depressed person goes through. It was left to me to reach out to him, take the initiative of calling him and engaging with him in longer conversations.

This is what a counsellor has to do to reach out to depressed people, more than in other cases, in order to build a rapport and relationship. This is particularly true in the initial phases of therapy because the depressed client is in a very passive state. More patience is required because the passivity and low energy, in some way, has to be compensated for by the counsellor. Very often, more information about the current situation has to be obtained from the caregivers and therefore, keeping in touch with them is also very important in such cases. Rushing any client in the process of counselling is not done but in the case of the depressed, one has to be extra watchful about the pace the counsellor is setting. There is a certain degree of constriction in their behaviour and pushing them to show progress just does not work and is likely to produce exactly the results the counsellor wants to avoid. In short, in the beginning, the process of counselling is a one way street from the counsellor to the client.

The depressed generally display a wide range of mood disorders. Their sleep pattern goes haywire and I have seen both types of eating disorders – mindless gluttony on one end of the scale and total lack of interest in food on the other. They tend to spend time in bed and despite that, complain of fatigue. The long winter nights aggravates the illness. Since some cases are genetically caused, it is a good idea to check whether any other member of the family has a depressive disposition. In very mild cases of depression, bordering on sadness

Put some Sense into this Boy's Head

and blues, aerobic exercises are known to help.

Counsellors are likely to become stressed when dealing with such cases and they need to share their own thoughts and feelings about the client by talking to someone in a similar profession. Remember it will be a slow process. Though not visible, progress is taking place.

I must repeat this because evaluation by a psychiatrist is of utmost importance. The lead role is that of the doctor. The supporting role belongs to the counsellor.

When we are in relationship with the client and they tell us something is going on, they also give us major clues on what is going on.

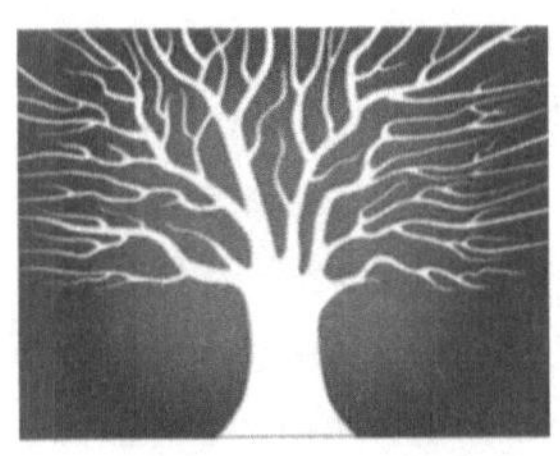

Marriage is about love; divorce is about money. ~ Anonymous

An acquaintance of mine called to say his niece's marriage was in trouble and asked if I could help the couple resolve their differences. When we met, the couple said they had been married for five years but their relationship was cold and the erotic passion one would expect in the early days of marriage was missing. I asked them to start at the beginning of their marriage and this is what came out, mostly from the husband, Arvind. The wife, Usha, left the narration to her husband.

Arvind was an IT professional and theirs was an arranged marriage. They met for the first time at Usha's house in Mysore, where her father was then posted. Following a couple of meetings between the two sets of parents and the couple, the decision to get married was taken; the proverbial nuptial knot was tied and the bride moved to Bangalore to live with her husband and his parents. They described their marriage as an 'arranged love marriage', a description I was not previously aware of.

The husband then stated that the marriage was not working for them overall. When queried about details, the following narrative unfolded over three or four sessions: Usha would routinely emerge from her room an hour after Arvind had left for work in the morning, dressed for the day. She then had tea and breakfast served by the mother-in-law, took a short walk around the house and then went back to her room to rest. She mostly stayed in the room, with minimal contact with her parents-in-law. Their hope was that after settling down, their daughter-in-law would take over the household chores like buying the groceries, or planning the day's meals; that she would eat

This one ended in Divorce

with them. But after a few months, they found nothing of this sort happened. It appeared that Usha spent the whole day quite happily by herself, doing nothing but watching TV or changing dresses and make-up. Sometimes she would go to a nearby park, walk a bit and sit on a bench, and then return. It was 'hi' and 'bye' contact with her in-laws. She seemed to have little desire to get to know her husband's family better or to make new friends in the locality. This disappointed Arvind's parents and they began to mention it to their son, who asked them to give her more time. However, nothing changed substantially month after month, year after year.

The only thing that seemed to interest the young bride was new clothes and make-up. She would spend a disproportionate amount of time looking at herself in the mirror and trying different shades of make-up. Even I noticed this habit; she would take out a hand mirror from her bag, do up her hair and face, and adjust her clothing before she walked in for counselling. Arvind kept telling his parents to give her more time to adjust, but 'how much more?' was their question. Whenever Arvind raised the issue with Usha, she told him that she had no interest in household chores.

Arvind found this disturbing, as also her coldness in the bedroom when he tried to initiate sex. "Not now, we will do it tomorrow," was her usual response; and if he did succeed, there were lukewarm responses. He took Usha for holidays to faraway places, hill stations, beaches and resorts – hoping that romantic settings would trigger romantic responses from her. But the romantic return on investments made by the husband in time and money remained woefully low. Whenever they were out together, Usha was only interested in visiting malls, window shopping (which she could do for hours), and buying new clothes.

Hindi songs like *Too hi toh meri jannat ho* (You are my heaven, you are my earth) perpetuate the belief that this is what love is all about. But what these songs and dancing around trees in hill stations represent

This one ended in Divorce

is infatuation, not love. It is not by changing the geographical location of your bed that love suddenly appears. In love, you do not become a doormat, and let your lover walk all over you. Love is hard work.

Arvind, after waiting for nearly five years for things to change, decided to call it quits and declared his intentions to his and her parents. Usha would return to her parents' house. The hope in both families was that the separation would do her good and she would long to be reunited with he husband. Separation did produce temporary results in that she would ring up and ask Arvind to take her back home to start a new innings; but soon things would be back to square one.

Now to Usha's version of the marriage. She made it sound that what Arvind and his parents were saying was no big deal and she did not understand why he was in such a great hurry. "Things will work out only if Arvind is more patient – he is so impatient!" she complained to me. On the sexual aspect of her marriage, there were two answers: one, that Arvind did not know how to excite her; and the second, that he was always in a hurry. Usha came across as a person who felt that a big mountain was being made out of a molehill. Easy does it was her view. Arvind felt that he could wait no longer because if he had to make another life (a second go at marriage); he could not wait until he was getting dentures.

I should have mentioned that after a fortnight of contact with me, Usha's parents also came to see me. What her father revealed gave a significant clue to Usha's behaviour. He said, "I now think that I should have been stricter with Usha. I loved her so much that I would do anything for her. Her every little wish was a command for me. I couldn't see the little one cry. My heart would melt when she asked for something, whether it was a certain type of chocolate or a dress. She just had to ask for something and I would drop everything and happily do it, even if I had just come home tired. I now wonder whether my treatment of her made her too soft. I don't know. I am confused. But I am sure you will solve the problem and they will stay married.

This one ended in Divorce

Otherwise it will be a great shock to us and our reputation in society will be mud."

Some readers will be familiar with the marshmallow experiment that psychologists have done with young children. Children were given two choices: either to get one marshmallow immediately, or get two marshmallows after an hour. The results showed that while two-thirds of the children could not wait and opted for instant gratification, a third of them preferred to wait for better options later. Usha got all the marshmallows immediately all the time and so instant gratification became a habit.

Her mother had this to say: "I kept telling him that he was spoiling Usha. She would get away with anything. She needed discipline, but he wouldn't listen. He could not bear to see his daughter crying. I think Arvind is right. She is acting spoilt with him and her in-laws. But I am sure that you will put some sense into her head and she will not act so spoilt." Most parents think the counsellor has a magic wand that will erase the scars of their dear ones. What they do not perceive is that for a person to change, he has to change internally.

Readers will recall how in one of the previously cited case studies on attempted suicide, the person was mauled in childhood, criticised, compared and condemned by her parents. She thought it was not worth living and the pain of living was so much that she wanted to end it by dying. This question must surely arise in your minds: why do parents do this? The answer is simple. There is no profession in the world that you can practice for a lifetime, without any training. Can you be a teacher? No. Can you be a lawyer without training? Can you join an infotech company without any formal training? No way. However, the most important role in the world – parenting – can be entered into without training because after all, we see it being practiced by our parents. Our parents may have made a mess of parenting because they saw their parents do it that way. And so the rotten arm of parenting extends from generation to generation.

This one ended in Divorce

Someone has wisely said that we are 'victims of victims'. Our parents were victims of poor parenting and we do the same thing to our children and produce more victims.

It was my impression that Usha's father did exactly that – out of love but also ignorance – by giving in to all of her demands, big or small. This approach is called engulfment. You engulf the child in your arms and do everything for it, so that the child grows up believing the whole world will be waiting on them, to meet their wishes. And when they discover the world is too busy to give them even a second look, they come crashing down. As much as the three Cs (criticism, comparison and condemnation) in childhood have adverse effects in adulthood, so does engulfment.

The polar opposite of engulfment is disciplining children in an indisciplined way, by slapping, kicking or punching them. In my view, the worst abusive form of indisciplined discipline is when parents do not walk the talk to their children, or when they give lengthy lectures on good behaviour (for example, the child should not throw tantrums), but their own behaviour with each other is subject to tantrums. On the other hand, if children find their parents live disciplined lives and keep the promises they make, those attributes become part of the DNA of the children as well.

Since parenting is a subject talked about so sparingly, it needs more space here. An infant, at the time of birth, is helpless and has no identity. Its identity is closely tied up with that of the parents, particularly that of the mother, who breastfeeds it. In fact, the mother and child have what philosophers call a symbiotic relationship. They are two but perceive each other as one. As the infant grows, he begins to see some boundaries: 'I am I, and my brother is my brother'. Over time, he begins to see himself as a being who is separate from his brother. However, he is still hugely dependent on his parents. At this stage, the child has no knowledge of God, values, right or wrong. The parents are God. What they do becomes the child's model of doing. If they say that he

This one ended in Divorce

should tell visitors they are not home when, in fact, they are, he learns it is a perfectly legitimate way of getting out of a tricky situation. If he is mollycoddled as Usha was in childhood, mollycoddling is what he expects when he grows up, for that was the only mode he was exposed to. That becomes the compass, the direction of his life.

Now the reader will see why Usha acted in the way she did. If parents continue to treat their children as children, even when they have grown up, they keep them in a state of dependency. That is why there was no initiative on Usha's part to go out and buy groceries, make contact with others in the neighbourhood, or take the initiative in cooking. Right from childhood things were done for her. It is thus a parental duty to move children from dependency to independence, by letting them manage their own lives as they grow up. It is only when they have tasted independence that they can move to the next stage – interdependence. They cannot jump there without first being independent. This could have been Usha's problem. She was, in psychological terms, still a child.

Does it mean that once this way, always this way? There are no simple answers. Some see the light when the world gives them frequent kicks in the backside; some gain insights through counselling; and some wake up on their own. That some do get insights on their own is revealed by the following case study reported by social scientists: There was a father who was in and out of jail, graduating from petty crimes to bigger ones, then moving on to even more serious and heinous ones. He had two sons, one of whom also went to jail. When the authorities profiled him, they found that he too, had literally taken the same path as his father, moving from small infringements to gory crimes. They asked him the reason for his life's story. He summed it up in a one-liner: "With a father like mine, what else could I be?"

From this brother, the authorities got to know the whereabouts of the other brother and located him. They found he was a dentist, happily married, the proud father of two children. They asked him how he had

This one ended in Divorce

shaped his life so differently from his brother and were shocked when he said the same thing his brother had: "With a father like that, what else could I be?" Fullstop. I leave no insights here – please draw your own conclusions.

Getting back to Usha and Arvind, I would see the couple together as well as separately. This is often necessary for two reasons. The basis of the issues being dealt with are often different, and the pace at which each person makes changes is different too. In the combined sessions, I asked the couple to come out with their expectations about each other. Unexpressed expectations are great spoilers in marriage. Often the expectations of one partner are unreasonable, or not even stated (it is assumed the partner should know). So, in marital counselling, it is very important for partners to lay bare their expectations and negotiate what is possible and what is not. Once accepted, they have to try and meet those expectations.

In the case of this couple, Usha would agree to try to help her mother-in-law and perform her conjugal duties. But not much progress would be made week after week. Usha's position was that she be given more time as, "I have been telling you Uncle, Arvind expects too much from me, too soon." After some sessions, I met the couple together and told them there was little more I could do to help them. The time had come for them to take a position on the future of their marriage. Arvind was clear he would wait no longer and preferred divorce and a new beginning elsewhere.

When asked my opinion on divorce, I said that when things do not work out, as seemed to be the case here, divorce was a legitimate culmination of the counselling process. Hearing this, Usha burst into tears. I think she saw it as a big rejection – something she had not experienced before. But if all efforts to save a marriage fails, disengagement through divorce is best not only for the two partners but also for the children of the marriage. The counselling process stopped for Arvind and Usha. I eventually heard they had divorced.

This one ended in Divorce

Coming back to the topic of parenting, there is another issue that needs mentioning, called abandonment. Let me give you an example. The father is reading a newspaper and his six-year-old son tries to draw his attention to something that happened at school. The father continues to read the paper but tells the son, "Carry on. Why have you stopped? I am listening to you." The child, young as he may be, is smart enough to think, "I am not worth my father's complete attention". He may forget it once or twice. But if he finds a pattern in this kind of response, he begins to see himself as a person of low worth, and in some cases, carries that image into adulthood.

Take another example. The father promises that when he returns from work and after an early dinner, he will take the children out for ice cream. If he breaks his promises once too often, his children grow up with the worldview: 'Can I trust these people? After all, my father said so many things he did not mean. I'd better watch out.' So, as parents, we must be careful to be role models of the values we want our children to imbibe. It is not through lectures and sermons that we pass on our message. It is through our behaviour and its consistency that we can create their worldview. Parenting is a serious role. What is covered here is just an overview. If opportunities come your way to learn more about parenting, do grab them. Meanwhile, you may want to pay heed to these wise words:

I don't love him because he is good but because he is my child.
– Rabindranath Tagore

The hardest part of raising a child is teaching him to ride bicycles. A shaky child on a bicycle for the first time needs both freedom and support. The realization that this is what the child will always need, can hit hard.
– Sloan Wilson

Love is the chain whereby to bind a child to its parents. – Anon

This one ended in Divorce

GURUSPEAK: MARRIAGE COUNSELLING

Counselling the depressed is a difficult process. Marital counselling, married counsellors believe, is easy because, being married ourselves, we believe we are aware of the dynamics of marriage and the intricacies involved. Our own marriages may be messy but we have QED solutions for others. Instead, this is what counsellors need to do.

It is difficult enough to deal with the issues of one person but to deal with those of two, does not mean the issues become two dimensional. On the contrary, they become multi-dimensional. Bring in the children and the families of the unhappy couple and the other stakeholders, and you have a mountain of issues to deal with. In marriage counselling, many of the counsellor's personal prejudices often creep in, such as: This is not the way for the wife to behave. The husband should provide more space to his wife for her to grow. Other personal *shoulds* can infect the counselling process. One of the recommended approaches is that the cousellor shun personal prejudices before entering the counselling room and be constantly aware of his own prejudices intruding on the narrative.

It is my experience that in marital counselling, the wife is usually more emotional in expressing her pain and disappointment. The husband might give the impression of being stoic, although deep inside, he too, is burning. But the crying, emotionally-charged wife may tip the balance of counselling in her favour. In marital counselling, each partner tries to get their point of view across. The more articulate a partner is in conveying a context that suits them, the greater the chance of the counsellor feeling anger towards the other.

It has been observed that counsellors can fall into the trap of perceiving one party as being in the right and the other in the wrong. Awareness, awareness, awareness is the key. It is for the counsellor to give equal space to both, ensuring that he alone poses questions to both partners and does not permit personal attacks and counterattacks between the two. The atmosphere in the room can get totally vitiated and charged if civility is given the go by. Therefore, I suggest that the earlier sessions are best conducted individually, to first build equal comfort levels with both partners before joint sessions are launched.

Another important point in marital counselling, and perhaps in all counselling, is that our own value systems should not become the filter through which we engage with clients. The major issues that surface in marriage counselling are sex-related, control exercised by one upon the other or hidden escapades outside marriage. In India other areas of friction are the house budget, given to the wife by the husband, and physical and verbal abuse. We have to remember that in marriage there are two humans behind any issue and disharmony – we must focus on the two individuals and not just on the problem.

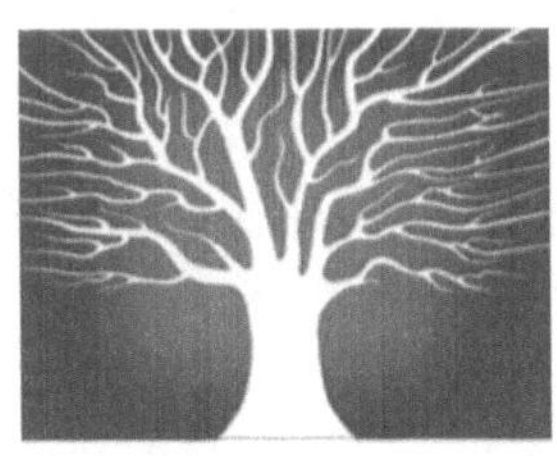

Does the question, 'What has counselling got to do with seasickness?' come to mind? In a particular context it does – when dealing with issues of adolescence, the choppiest period in life, a period of confusion, rebellion and peer pressure. It is also a time of confusion because you do not know whether you are a girl or a woman; a boy or a man; dependent or independent; whether you can decide or your parents should. A wise person has likened adolescence to a traveller on a ship sailing choppy waters on the high sea. He feels sick and vomits. But when the seas become calm, he can even laugh at the experience.

This is the case of an adolescent. The parents, in their mid-forties, walked in with their teenage son. When they had sat down and seemed about to begin their verbal assault on the handsome boy, I asked them to wait while I found a comfortable place for him to sit outside the chamber. I have now made this my routine when I get a whiff about parents bringing their charges of correction to me. Why? Because, one too many times, I have witnessed the young ones being demolished by parents in the presence of a total stranger – myself. Very often, I have sensed the underlying causes were the parents.

There is another reason why I believe youngsters need support from me. Not just because they are young, but in most cases, they do not say anything to let down their parents, even when minutes before, the parents may have badmouthed them. On numerous occasions I have got "Fine" as a response when I queried them about how things were going between them and their parents. So I not only take them out to make them feel comfortable but also assure them I will listen to their parents and then spend a lot of time with them to understand their

A case of Seasickness

side of the story. I also assure them that just because I am seeing the parents first, it does not mean I am giving them priority or preference but because they have come to me first. This is a very important aspect of counselling. Imagine waiting outside when your parent is being seen first by the counsellor – you begin visualising yourself being declared guilty before you have a chance to speak to the counsellor. You are bound to experience the second person syndrome.

On returning to the room, I asked the parents the issue that had brought them to me. They said they had no problem but their son did (another fact of counselling is that it is mostly the other person who has a problem). They had this to say: Their son Naresh was their older child. They had a daughter who was three years younger. Until a year ago, all was hunky dory with Naresh. He was a well-behaved boy, a good student, he had got along well with friends, and there was nothing to complain about. However, things changed drastically in the last year. Naresh's grades slipped, he came home late, missed classes, and the school warned the parents that Naresh would have to mend his ways or he would be expelled. They were at their wit's end to know why his behaviour had deteriorated so much. He would not listen to any advice from them and instead, took an aggressive position to defend himself, accusing his teachers of bias, and pretending he was fine but the others were not. Naresh would get angry if his demands for a superior cell phone were not met or he was told to tidy up his room.

The more they revealed, the more I got into a *filmi* style flashback of my own life. I am tempted to narrate this because everything that was happening to Naresh had happened to me when I was fifteen, sixty years ago, except that there were no cell phones, hardly any landlines, or cars where I lived in the early 1950s. Let me start with a pat on the back. A serious learner, always doing my assignments, 100% attendance and good reports from school, was my track record until the pre-matriculation period (10th standard of today); and until Ram Swaroop and I became good friends. He became my hero and I blindly followed everything he did. That meant bunking classes,

A case of Seasickness

seeing movies on the sly, telling lies to my parents to get out of tricky situations, slipping up on homework, coming home late – in short, doing everything that was not supposed to be done. Suddenly a 'good' boy called Dinesh became the 'bad' boy Dinesh. Well-deserved thrashings, curfews, pocket money cuts, and 'this-way-you-will-not-get-anywhere' warnings followed. The more I got them, the more I retaliated through rebellious responses. My younger brother, who has a sharp memory, now makes fun of me by telling my children and grandchildren how I would slip out of bed to see late night movies after my parents had gone to sleep. Then, as suddenly as I had become a 'bad' boy, I once again became a 'good' boy. I did not know then but I do now, that I had an extreme case of seasickness called adolescence.

Fast-forwarding to the present, I saw Naresh after I had finished talking to his parents. He had nothing much to say except, "Yeah, my grades have come down but I am trying hard. But nobody believes me. Everybody thinks I am not paying attention. I keep fooling around, they say, but that is not true. My parents get all worked up about little things. I can't do anything right according to them." To every, "What else?" from me, his response was that he did not have anything more to say. It did not take me long to conclude that his case was not much different from mine all those years ago. Naresh was going through seasickness. Soon, just as I became a 'good' boy, he too, would become a 'good' boy.

Let us look at some issues connected with adolescence. Whenever I have to do a parenting workshop, at the beginning of the programme connected with how to deal with adolescent children, I take great pleasure in saying: "Children of today love luxury. They have bad manners and love to chatter. They no longer rise when elders enter the room. They contradict their parents, gobble up the dainties at the table and are tyrants over their teachers." I see the parents vigorously nodding their heads in agreement; and then I ask, "True, isn't it?" Their responses convey total agreement. I pause and then break the news that this is what a Greek philosopher said 2500 years ago. I tell them that the generation gap existed even then. Perhaps the gap has increased even more now. If we parents do not move with the times and start understanding the issues involved with adolescence, we have only ourselves to blame.

It was clear that Naresh's parents needed to be told some facts about adolescent behaviour and to be reassured that Naresh would get over it. Also, they had to know that controlling Naresh's behaviour would not work. It would only serve to drive him away from them. Here are some of the things I shared with them over the next few sessions: I acknowledged their feelings were real and every generation of parents has thought similarly. However, they needed to be aware that the context in which they were brought up was different and if they tried to superimpose their contextual ethos on the current framework, it would just not work. If they believed that what applied in their day should apply in the days of internet and mobile telephony, they were not being fair. Today, people live in a globalised world and this generation is exposed to many more influences than before. Therefore, if adolescents grow or dye their hair, do not make a big deal of it – they will grow out of it. Their personality content is not tied up with the colour of their hair.

I told them that even the WHO has segmented adolescence into the age group of ten to twenty years, for us to understand there are be behavioural changes. And there are rapid physical changes too, which sometimes confuse teenagers and traumatise them. Imagine the shock when a young girl first starts menstruating or a boy has wet dreams. Will there not be confusion in their minds which they cannot handle? Their emotions are at a peak and if we do not realise this, then conflicts are bound to emerge. Understanding their emotional issues, rather than challenging them, is the best way to deal with them. Otherwise, we can end by driving them up the wall towards taking drugs, smoking and drinking. As it is, in today's world there is tremendous peer pressure to try drugs or alcohol.

The other thing I told Naresh's parents was that there is so much

A case of Seasickness

confusion at this age because youngsters cannot get a clear fix on who they are – child or adult, dependent or independent – and these conflicts lead them to behave irrationally by missing classes or leaving their rooms in a chaotic state. I asked Naresh's parents whether all the controls they had tried to impose on him had worked. They replied in the negative. I then suggested they could set some limits on behaviour but keeping a messy room should not be made into a big deal. "Become Naresh's friends and stop parenting him," was another insight I left behind in one of the sessions. I have read, and it made a lot of sense to me, that youngsters complain that when they are growing up, their parents stop growing; they become stuck, treating them like little children, which they no longer are.

We need to realise that their peers are everything to adolescents, but not for us adults. Their world revolves around their peers and not around us. As adults we must remember that these changes are temporary and show patience. Going along with the flow of their growth is a better way of dealing with them than resisting. Yes, Naresh's grades had fallen and that was a matter of concern; but to call him stupid was driving him away; and if he wanted to be left alone, he had to be given that space.

When I talk to youngsters as equals, they tell me their parents have become big time nosy parkers, wanting to know everything, interfering in everything, controlling, and critical of their friends. "They want to hear every word we say on the phone but they don't know that we can fool them in our own way." Control, control and more control. When that does not work, criticising, calling teens stupid, comparing and demeaning them, are some methods parents resort to – which only serves to drive them away.

Parents have to make a choice: would you rather let your son keep his room messy for a couple of years or have marathon arguments with him and drive him out of a bonded relationship that took so long to build? Would you rather sermonise on smoking and taking drugs or enter into communication with openers like what he thinks of smoking and drugs? Communication takes effort but sermonising is a lazy way out. Most parents take the lazy way, not because they are indifferent towards their children but because they did not take the time to learn a few things about parenting, believing they knew all about it.

Also, let us remind ourselves that we live in the age of 'Hi dude', 'I'm good' and 'Cool', and not in our world of 'How do you do?' and "I'm fine, thank you'. I can't think of better advice than to quote Khalil Gibran's advice to parents in his book, *The Prophet*.

Your children are not your children.
They are the sons and daughters of life's longing for itself.
They come through you but not from you,
And though they are with you, yet they belong not to you.
You may give them your love but not their thoughts
For they have their own thoughts.
You may house their bodies but not their souls,
For their souls dwell in the house of to-morrow, which you cannot visit, not even in your dreams.
You may strive to be like them, but seek not to make them like you. For life goes not backward nor tarries with yesterday.
You are the bows from which your children as living arrows are sent forth.
The archer sees the mark upon the path of the infinite, and He bends you with His might that His arrows may go swift and far.
Let your bending in the archer's hand be for gladness.
For even as He loves the arrow that flies, so He loves also the bow that is stable.

Fortunately for Naresh, his parents were open to suggestions and willing to see the world from his viewpoint. A couple of counselling sessions were enough for them to understand the issues involved with adolescence and the ways of dealing with them.

While Naresh's issue was resolved because his parents saw some sense in what I was telling them, more often than not, parents continue with control psychology. But the more they resist the behaviour of the young, the more the young persist with their behaviour. The choices parents make are certainly in their domain, but when it comes to facing the consequences that follow those choices, they often pay in terms of the cost of an unhappy relationship with their very own.

In adolescence, stop being a parent and become a friend to your children. If there is one thing children recall, years later, it is how they were treated during this phase.

GURUSPEAK: ADOLESCENCE

A few insights that a counsellor can provide to parents with adolescent children are: It is best to accept this phase as a reality and not resist it. You will see restlessness in them and that they want to wean away from parental control and supervision. Why? Because they are seeking the kind of independence they truly deserve. And look at the larger picture of the relationship between parents and youngsters. Conversing with them, offering insights and suggestions during the course of dialogues, in which the young ones see parents as equal partners, works better than confronting them. Let me quote what many adolescents have told me: 'Who the hell cares if my room is messy? I am living there. What is the big deal?' Frankly, I agree.

Other insights parents could bear in mind: Avoid saying 'It serves you right, I have been telling you, it will not work for you but you just don't listen.' If the issue is critical, it is best to give reasons for your concern. One thing adolescents do not like at all and can take umbrage to is having their privacy invaded. In critical areas, parents need to set non-negotiable boundaries and be consistent in enforcing them. Once that is done, children are discerning enough to know the no-no areas.

There are a few other pointers that counsellors can suggest to parents. The most important is not to try and realize their own unrealized ambitions through the lives of their children; do not try to make your son an engineer because you wanted to be one but could not make it.

A case of Seasickness

It is the experience of many counsellors that when the atmosphere in a home is full of negativity, then to expect a child to be blazing positivity, is to ask for too much.

The last thing that I must mention here is that parents must keep the doors of communication open. Shutting the door and being inflexible can only cause serious relationship ruptures and parents can lose their children for life at an emotional level.

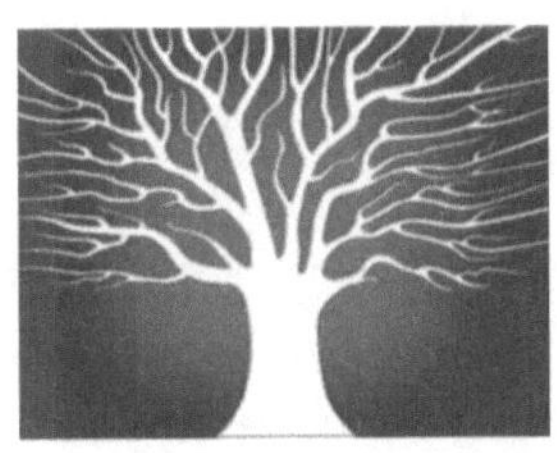

Child abuse casts a shadow the length of a lifetime. ~ Herbert Ward

If an ad-man was looking for a made-for-each-other couple, Azhar and Anjali would have won hands down. A more graceful or handsome pair I had not met before. They had a certain presence whenever they came into the room to meet me. They were both articulate, considerate and well mannered. Love was written all over their faces, yet they had been dealing with a personal issue for the last five years.

Azhar and Anjali had met in a gym. Both were fitness freaks, with an eye constantly on their body mass index. After workouts, they would chat over energy drinks. One thing led to another and soon they were deeply in love. That they belonged to different religions was not something that bothered them. In one of our sessions, when the subject of inter-religion marriages and the difficulties associated with them cropped up, their view was to let those who had these issues resolve them; it was not for them to carry someone else's baggage.

So what was the issue they were dealing with? Although they had been married for five years, their marriage had still not been consummated. When it came to giving more details, Azhar asked to speak to me alone and Anjali had no issue with that. Azhar told me they loved each other deeply and nothing had changed, but when it came to having sex, Anjali would freeze and become frigid. There were times, Azhar said, when she would run out of bed, lock herself in the bathroom and cry and cry. Then, from sheer exhaustion, she would return and sleep. Azhar showed her all the patience he could and believed that perhaps Anjali needed more time. There was no bashing, no blame game between them, despite the fact that they were dealing with a

In Love but cannot Make Love

serious marital issue. One day, over the dinner table, they discussed the issue like two responsible people and decided to seek counselling help. That was what brought them to me.

In my first session, I asked the question that needed to be asked: whether in her early childhood, Anjali had been sexually abused. Unlike in other similar cases, where people who have been abused in their childhood tend to deny the fact and wipe it from their psyche, Anjali's answer was in the affirmative. This is what she told me: Anjali lived with her parents in a large upmarket housing complex and their neighbours on the same floor were her uncle and aunt. Often, when she was only five, her parents would leave her with them when they went out for social events in the evening or out of town for the weekend.

One day, her uncle came to her room while she was lying down and started talking to her about school. He offered her chocolates and then starting touching her private parts and even forcing himself on her. After this assault, he threatened her with dire consequences if she mentioned a word of what had happened. "Do you understand?" he asked and he would accept only an affirmative answer. He then gave her some chocolates, kissed her and smooched around for some time. This carried on for almost a year. Anjali was too scared of the consequences and kept her hurt to herself, until she could no longer bear the burden of the frequent assaults not only on her body but also on her dignity. She felt traumatised before, during and after the episodes, until one day she felt enough was enough and confided in her mother.

She was shocked and taken aback by her mother's response. Anjali was slapped and accused of behaving badly and inciting her uncle to unbecoming behaviour. Her mother's command was no different from her uncle's: "Don't you dare open your mouth unless you want to be locked up in your room, you silly girl! You will bring shame to the whole family if you mention anything against your uncle, who

In Love but cannot Make Love

is such a nice man and so fond of you." Anjali had no choice but to suffer in silence and live with the trauma she experienced at such a tender age.

Here, I must mention a few things about child abuse – a subject about which there is little said, but much needs to be discussed. The points below are presented in an abridged form.

Child abuse takes place in many forms, including verbal (thrashing the child with abusive language) and physical (thrashing the child physically and giving him scars and black eyes). But the worst form is sexual – the scars of which are the hardest to heal. This is one of the many societal issues that lies buried under the surface and needs to be brought out in the open, for general awareness. Indian society, mostly, is in a state of denial that a social problem like Child Sexual Abuse (CSA) actually exists. Therefore, even the shocking fact that such abuse occurs with every other girl and among one in six boys, is either not known or glossed over.

I now deal with some of the issues involving abused children and adults who were abused as children. If the abuse is currently going on, we must do all we can to stop it, which usually means taking the child out of the abusive situation. Most often, the abuse stops during childhood but surfaces later as the possible cause of adult problems. In many cases, children grow out of the abusive experience and learn to live normal lives; despite CSA experiences, they are still able to trust people. They have suffered but not been permanently damaged. However, in about 20% of cases, the trauma continues into adult life and has to be dealt with.

The aggressors in the case of child abuse, are usually people the child trusts. They include natural parents, uncles, cousins, neighbours and even teachers. The biggest casualty of such abuse is trust, when those who the child trusted the most become the abusers. Children do not know how to handle such a situation and therefore keep the experience

In Love but cannot Make Love

of abuse to themselves. They have little faith in the adult world and therefore buy peace by keeping mum.

In addition to the total loss of trust, CSA manifests itself in many other ways, like difficulty in entering into an intimate relationship, anxiety, depression, shame, guilt and anger. It is that shame and guilt, accompanied by a sense of entrapment, that keeps victims in a shell of misery, from which they find it difficult to break out, and the problem perpetuates. Survivors of CSA may either accidentally reveal the story or intentionally bring it to light because they want to learn how to deal with the painful and traumatic experience.

The worst thing we can do in these cases is to put the blame on the person concerned and say things like: 'It must have been your fault – you must have done something to encourage it. You are no good. Why did you allow such a thing to happen? Why did you not tell me this before?' This kind of response makes an already 'guilty' person feel even more ashamed. The other thing to remember is that most of us are not equipped to handle CSA cases by ourselves.

What parents need to do is to teach children what a good touch or a bad touch is, and how to deal with those who attempt to perpetrate this heinous crime on them. For example, by running away and shouting for help. Trust children. Keep telling them you trust them. If your child tells you about being sexually abused, you must believe the child, because a young one cannot make up an experience like that. They often have difficulty in even articulating their experience and just throw out a hint like, 'Uncle is bad'.

If the emotional scars continue to haunt the person, the only course of action is to seek counselling with an experienced person. During counselling, the survivors of CSA are made to see that they are not suffering so much from the abuse itself, as much as from the fact they have lost trust in people. In their experience, not trusting people makes sense to them. If they have been hurt by people who were their role

In Love but cannot Make Love

models, close relatives or neighbours, how can they possibly trust total strangers? What they need to learn is that most people are not abusers and most people – but not all – can be trusted. They have to learn to distinguish those who can be trusted from those who cannot, and stay clear of the second category. They have to be extra cautious to avoid being hurt again and lose what little trust they are beginning to gain.

There are two schools of thought in the counselling approach itself. One recommends revisiting the 'scene of crime' by talking about the abused history. This theory believes in going back in memory to create acceptance of that history. Personally, I do not see much merit in this approach and believe in the second approach, propagated by William Glassser, which says that everything we want to change is happening in the present, and revisiting a bad experience does not make the person any stronger. In his book, *Choice Theory*, Glasser puts it clearly, using a perfect analogy saying that if you have been starving for a long time, you need food, not an explanation why you were not fed in the past.

I believe that revisiting the past reinforces the script of negativity etched on one's neural circuits. The more we go into the past, the more the script is reinforced. I have tried this approach and personal experience tells me it takes a long time to resolve issues stemming from childhood scars. As someone once said, it is putting the person in an unresourceful state of mind and that can hardly produce resourceful results.

Whichever approach one takes in counselling, the belief remains that these psychological wounds can be healed through understanding and love; that trusting relationships can be built again. Admittedly, an abused person, because of an unhappy past, may be less capable, but not incapable, of dealing with the present. But that is true for all cases that enter the counselling process, regardless of the issue they are dealing with. The past does not interfere with the present unless we make the choice to live in the past. This needs to be emphasised to the survivors of abuse.

In Love but cannot Make Love

The idea is to replace the older clutter on the neural circuits with positive resourcefulness, by planting the thought that if the victim were not there at that point of time, the perpetrator would have done the heinous act to someone else any way; and thus remove the guilt from the mind of the person. Or by saying: 'You have had this awful experience, but are you going to give the power of your life to the useless perpetrator who may be enjoying a peg of scotch while you are wallowing in guilt? Take the power back into your hands. You deserve it. You are a unique gift to humanity and let no one, but no one, hijack your happiness.' In this way, we can open new neural circuits of resourceful positivity. If the song of pain comes back, push the button to the next song, a happy song.

As an aside, I might mention that studies done on the human brain have shown the following results:

- Those who are continuously engaged in new challenges expand the brain. For example, say you are sixty and have never played tennis before, and start learning the game. As you proceed, your brain has to create new neural circuits to help you respond to the serves, volleys and lobs you face on court. Your brain had never before dealt with such situations and has to learn new tricks by expanding to take on the new challenges.

- In real life, those who, regardless of age, choose to stay excited and have a what-next approach, seem to delay growing old. On the other hand, those who slide into retirement with no clear aim in life, tend to fade away. Anthony Robin, author of *Unlimited Power*, puts it in simple terms: 'Keep reprogramming your jukebox'.

What should the family or any other caregiver do when they accidentally or intentionally stumble upon a case of child abuse? The first and most important thing is to assure the child repeatedly that

In Love but cannot Make Love

it is not their fault and to reinforce your love and trust. Ensure the child is never again put into a situation where such abuse is possible, and look out for any behavioural pattern which indicates any of the effects mentioned above. In case something does come to your notice in the adulthood of the survivor, guide them to a reputed counselling centre. Do make a point to ask about the experience the counsellor has in dealing with such cases, for not all counsellors are trained to handle CSA. Asking for the credentials of the counsellor is your right and you must exercise it.

Brushing the issue of CSA under the carpet is not a solution. As I mentioned, the survivors of child sexual abuse lose trust. Their mind works like this: 'If my own uncle could do this to me, can I trust this adult whom I have just come to know?' Survivors, when they grow up and get into intimate relationships, go into freeze mode and say to themselves: 'Hang on, he will hurt me sexually. I cannot make the same mistake.' Their partners do not understand the drift that happens when the relationship matures to closeness. And one failure in love follows another. It is believed that in some cases, victims degrade and consider themselves as 'useless' objects, and offer themselves easily in successive sexual relationships. However, I admit I have not come across such a case personally.

Coming back to Anjali and Azhar, I asked Anjali whether she had shared her traumatic experience with Azhar. She said she had not seen any reason to, or she would have since there was nothing they did not share with each other – that was just the way they lived. I asked for her permission to share the information with Azhar in my next session with him. She readily agreed.

Anjali was a stable girl and so I decided to be direct in my approach to providing her with insights on CSA. I asked her to imagine that if she had not been placed with her uncle for safe custody when her parents were away from home, what he would have done to satisfy his lust. Her response, which reflected maturity, surprised me. She said she

In Love but cannot Make Love

was not sure but guessed he would perhaps have found someone else. "Exactly," I responded, emphatically explaining to her that an abuser is an abuser looking for victims. If her uncle had not done it to her, he would have done it to another child who was in his proximity. The chances were that she was not his only victim.

From the counselling point of view, it is important the client knows she was a victim of circumstances, and had no role whatsoever in the crime the abuser committed and perhaps continued to commit. I told Anjali that what she needed to remember was that her uncle was the guilty one and not she. It took a few sessions for her to overcome her doubts. However, there was another aspect that needed to be dealt with and that was the act of forgiving her uncle, and her mother, who had heaped accusations on her. Fortunately, Anjali was a loving and forgiving person and after six or seven sessions, she was able to put her past behind her.

In my brief sessions with Azhar, I kept him informed of the progress Anjali was making. I appreciated his contribution in giving unconditional love and support to Anjali. I slipped in the insight that of the two, his life was running well for him, so he could continue to be the backbone for Anjali. He said he would do whatever it took to help her. The happy conclusion was that I am on their guest list and look forward to spending an evening with them whenever invited.

The bounden duty of parents is to ensure their children are never put in circumstances where the possibility of child abuse exists. I personally believe we should take a better-safe-than-sorry approach. Teach children repeatedly what a good touch and a bad touch is. Advise them to scream for help and run out. Trust their word when they say anything about the abuse. Finally, ask yourself whether saving family face is more important than the child's future. If the survivor is told to remain silent and live with the pain, it also keeps the perpetrator on the loose, free to molest other children. The question is: Are we not then partners in crime?

In Love but cannot Make Love

GURUSPEAK: CHILD ABUSE

Counsellors should not be surprised if survivors of abuse grow up to be suspicious adults, because a lack of trust becomes a significant part of their personality. The scars are deep and the adverse effects of abuse can be enormous. This can affect the next generation because their internal dialogue is if it could happen to them, what stops it from happening to their children? They become overly watchful of their children's activities. A few of them even want to take revenge by abusing their own children when they grow up. Their self-esteem falls to such low depths that they start seeing themselves as objects of pleasure and even stop resisting moves on them, believing they deserve it. And they live lives full of guilt.

In the above mentioned case study, it was fortunate that Anjali's husband was an understanding person. In many cases, husbands sermonize that it is childish to continue to be affected by something that happened way back in childhood. Another important point to remember is that in case of married couples, the husband needs to be enrolled and educated on the aftermath of child sexual abuse. It also needs to be clarified that boys are not free from sexual assault, lest people think child abuse is limited to female children alone.

The last thing I would mention is that although the act is physical, its effect is emotional and needs to be resolved at the emotional level through understanding and reaching out. Building the client's self-esteem through positive strokes is something counsellors need to do for the survivor by constantly focusing on the message: If you were not present at the scene, the perpetrator would have abused someone else; therefore you are not the cause but an unfortunate victim.

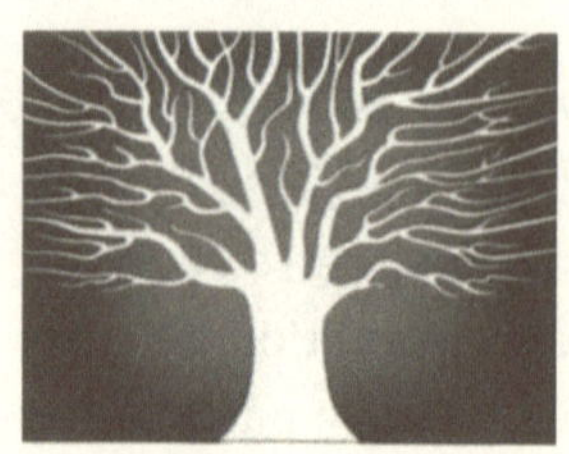

Immature love says: 'I love you because I need you.'
Mature love says: 'I need you because I love you.' ~ Erich Fromm

When counsellors meet informally to discuss issues of common interest, more often than not, the conclusion is that most of our cases stem from either relationship problems or low self-esteem. We readily agree that we are relating all the time to the people around us – family, colleagues and neighbours. And when we are not doing that, we are relating with ourselves, saying things like, 'Now that was a stupid thing to do' or 'I should not have said that'. We even relate to people who are not present: 'I put him in his place' or 'What does she think of herself?' or the awful traffic or weather: 'It is so hot'.

But what does all this have to do with playing rackets? I was attending an interactive workshop conducted by Landmark Education on life style issues. There were about 200 participants and as the programme progressed, they began sharing their experiences. The leader conducting the course would provide some insights into all the issues that came up during the discussions. In one session, a lady got up and said: "I have a younger brother who is very dear to me. I have looked after him as if he was my only child. His every wish was my command and I would do anything he asked. Then one day, I learnt that my brother had thrown a big party to celebrate his wedding anniversary. Many were invited but he did not call me. I was really mad at him. This was no way to treat me, I felt."

At this stage, she started sobbing. The leader went and stood beside her. Gently placing his arm around her shoulders, he gave her some tissues to wipe her tears and a glass of water. When she had regained her composure,

It is time to Stop Playing Rackets

he asked her to continue. She then narrated the subsequent part of her story, was punctuated by sobs and cries of anguish: "I stopped going to his house because I was very angry and felt let down. This was no way to treat a sister who had done so much for him. Then one day, I learnt he had suffered a massive heart attack and I felt I had to go and see him."

"What happened then?" asked the course leader.

"I got dressed to go," she continued, "but then the thought that my brother had not even had the courtesy to invite me to his anniversary party seemed too much to forget, and so I changed my mind."

There was pin drop silence in the hall. We could feel her anguish. The narration continued with the participant saying she heard from someone that her brother would be going to the UK for a heart surgery. She knew she had to go, not sure whether she would ever see him again. "I got into my car and headed towards the airport, but somewhere along the way I became angry again and was overwhelmed by a fit of rage. I told the driver to head back home."

We were all ears as she said in tears: "I came back home and prayed for his wellbeing. I kept saying to myself that I hope he would come back safe. Thank God, he did return safely. I am told he is improving but I still can't bring myself to put an end to my hurt and move on, having done all that I did for him all those years."

We were all with her in her pain. Then the leader walked back briskly towards centre stage and shouted at her: "Stop playing this silly racket game!" We almost rose in revolt at his insensitive remark, believing that here was a woman in so much pain, who was being shouted at. We felt that what he had done was utterly callous.

Then he dropped a big boulder, saying: "The only person who is standing between you and your brother is you yourself." He repeated the remark thrice, until it sank into our heads that in terms of relationship,

It is time to Stop Playing Rackets

we are the ones who hold back. We make the choice to hold back. He said he called this 'playing rackets', in which we are being someone or doing something but also complaining. Either we stop being that way and doing what we are doing, or we stop complaining. Which in this particular case meant, either disengaging with the brother and stop complaining, or engaging with him. He stopped short of saying that you can't have your cake and eat it too!

The course leader later explained what he termed the 'hurt to heal' philosophy, to provide an insight to all of us but most of all to the complaining sister. She got a breakthrough as the leader walked up to her and asked her to contact her brother and meet with him. She readily promised to do that. On being asked when, her response was that after the workshop was over she would make the first move. The leader gave another insight saying one should never wait to make the first move. "Do it now," he urged and sent her out of the hall to make the call to her brother.

She came back after a few minutes later to say he could not be contacted at that time. What followed the next day was heart-warming. The lady and her brother walked into the hall together, smiling, and made a public promise never to let niggardly things come in the way of important things like relationships. Hearing this, some others who were facing similar situations, declared that they would stop 'playing rackets'. If they could not do anything to mend relations, they would disengage; but they would stop complaining.

Many wise people have given insights on the subject of relationships and I recount some of them here. Stephen Covey, author of the bestselling book, *Seven Habits of Highly Effective People*, tells us that what others do or say is a stimulus we have no control over. The only control we have is over how we respond to it. He says we should make our choices with compassion, consciousness, awareness, independent will and imagination. Another piece of wise advice is: "For every miserable relationship, there is a huge pay off."

In the case of the lady and her brother, she was suffering, but that is not to say she was not getting a huge pay off in terms of ego, which translated meant: 'What does my brother think of himself? This is no way to behave with his elder sister. He must pay a reasonable return on the investment in time that I spent on him.'

Psychiatrist William Glasser says that we choose to be miserable and that every miserable relationship points to these four possibilities:

- That you are trying to dominate someone and it is not working for you.
- Someone is trying to dominate you and you don't like it.
- Both these things are happening simultaneously.
- You are doing something that you don't like doing.

Check yourself against the following statements:
'Your relationships with others are a mere reflection of your relationship with your parents.'
'If your relationship with yourself is not happy, it is unlikely that you will have happy relationships with others. '

Now mull over the next statement for five minutes: 'Relationships go sour because they were entered into for the wrong reasons'. Let us say you had an agenda in your mind to enter into a relationship and you did not succeed. You will be disappointed, but you also need to ask yourself what gave you the right to set the agenda? Did the other person know what you had in mind? Did the other person agree to it? This happens more and more in marital relationships. A horde of expectations from partners translate into heaps of disappointment when they are not met, and then the blame game starts. The most successful marriages are those where partners give free space to each other to grow and follow their own pursuits.

'The purpose of a relationship is not to have another who might complete you but to have another with whom you can share your completeness.' This wise statement will take some time to sink in but its efficacy cannot be disputed.

It is time to Stop Playing Rackets

'It is not in the action of another but in your reaction that your salvation would be found.' This is similar to Stephen Covey's words – that we have no control whatsoever on what others will do or say. The only thing that we can control is our response to others.

The next few statements are there for us to reflect on and see what we understand from them; also how we can apply them in our day-to-day lives. The next time we experience an unhappy situation in a relationship, the chances are that some rules of the game were violated.

- Relinquish your need to be right.
- Allow space for others to grow.
- Eliminate the idea of ownership.
- Know that you don't have to understand.
- The source of relationship problems is not 'out there' but 'in here'.
- Miserable relations are unmet expectations.
- Don 't sweat the small stuff; it is all small stuff.
- You cannot relate with others unless you can relate with yourself.
- The only person whose behaviour we can control is our own.
- Dysfunctional relationships often mean a dysfunctional relationship with oneself.
- A basic truth about relationships is that we chose to set them up this way.
- More judgmental the attitude, worse the relationships.
- Larger the expectations, more the issues in relationships.
- Like yourself before liking others.
- If good relationships are nurtured, so are poor relationships.
- Ask: What am I doing or not doing to have poor relationships?
- Ask not: What are others doing or failing to do in relationships?
- It is when we change that others change?
- We often want more than we are willing to give.
- Good relationships require hard work, like good health.
- At least admit I am one half of the deal.
- In the car journey of a relationship, we are at the steering wheel.
- A relationship is a risky business.

It is time to Stop Playing Rackets

◎◎ Self-righteousness is the biggest killer of relationships.
◎◎ Ask what Love requires me to do now.

The last bit of advice comes from none other than the spiritual leader Osho, who declared: "The other is hell". Which other was he talking about – the mother other, the father other, the neighbour other, the friend other, the boss other or the colleague other? What the wise man pointed out was that we will live in a veritable hell if we wait for the proper behaviour of others for our happiness. He then asks us to assume for a moment that we have sorted out the mother; then the father's behaviour might come into play. Assume we have sorted both out; then the neighbour might throw a tantrum, and so on. Do not get into the vicious circle of sorting out others. Sort out our own behaviour. In a relationship, when we have tried our best and things still do not work, disengaging from that person is the best policy.

Let us never forget that when we live in this world, we are bound with relationships. In that, we have no choice. The only choice we have is how we choose to relate with our family, friends, marriage, work and neighbourhood.
~ Unknown

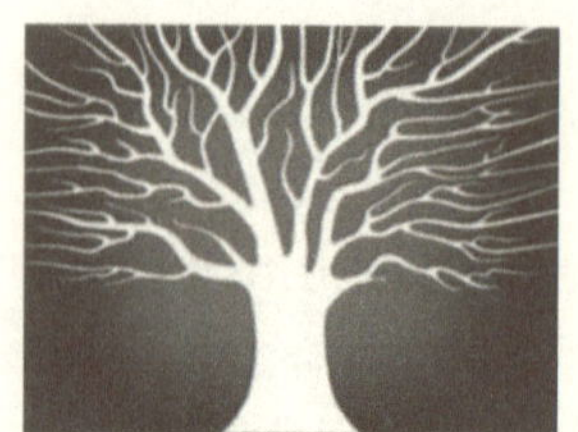

Part I: Cases & Consequences

YES DARLING, NO DARLING, HELLO DARLING

The one who loves least controls the relationship. ~ Robert Newton Anthony

This is how Arun Lal Gupta, a successful trader in auto parts, would address his wife Kiran, at social gatherings with his friends. But the inside story, narrated to me by Kiran herself, was different. She had been married to Arun for thirty years before she came to me for counselling. She had lived in an abusive marriage from day one. Yes, from day one. Although she came from an educated family, the family was rooted in the traditional view of marriage in which the husband called the shots and the in-laws could get away with just about anything.

Kiran was just a day-old bride when she was rudely summoned by her mother-in-law, who was lying in bed. The mother-in-law directed her to massage her legs, which needed warming up before she could get out of bed. Kiran did what she was asked to, while the MIL gave a running commentary on how her parents had not even taught her how to massage properly. Finally, the MIL kicked Kiran hard on her arms to indicate she should stop. She then told her the chores she was required to perform during the day. Initially Kiran did not mention this to Arun but after a few days of doing the early morning massage, she did pick up the courage to mention, very docilely, the treatment she was receiving from her MIL. Her husband's response shocked her: "What is the big deal, you stupid woman? Don't come running to me for these stupid things. Learn to live with my mother, okay?" And thus their marriage started on a platform of abuse.

It was after thirty years of living in an abusive marriage, which had all the three ingredients of physical, verbal and sexual abuse, that Kiran came to me. She was treated like an object rather than a living

Yes Darling, No Darling, Hello Darling

human being. Every little decision was taken by the husband and that included which curtains to buy for the house and which saree she should wear for a party. On the way to friends homes for dinner, there would be no conversation between the two except for some brutal criticism of Kiran and regret at having married a dunce of a woman. However, for public consumption, "no darling", "yes darling" and "hello darling" would start as the party progressed and alcohol took charge of Arun, a big time drinker. Her self-esteem was in the pits, having been eroded bit by bit – so much so that she began to accept this as a way of life to which there was no other alternative. When she described her horrible situation to her parents, 'adjust' was the only word she received in response. And in these thirty years, she had borne two daughters and one son.

I mentioned that she had been reduced to a mere object. On the family's annual excursions with Arun's three brothers and their families, the youngest brother, his spirits buoyed by spirits imbibed through the evening, would touch her body in an indecent manner, with not a word of protest from her husband. Arun would laugh and call his brother a naughty boy. During one such trip, this brother entered her bedroom when she was alone and started kissing and hugging her. Arun assumed she must have done something to invite his brother's attentions since his brother would never otherwise stoop so low. The more she got this kind of treatment, the more used Kiran became to it. It was like the experiment in which you dip your hand into lukewarm water and the temperature is increased gradually; your hand gets used to the incremental change and is not not withdrawn even when the water becomes hot. Kiran accepted this was her fate.

The narration about her marriage continued over many sessions I had with her. The flirtatious behaviour did not start and end with her brother-in-law; it extended to one of Arun's friends, who treated his wife not much differently than Arun did his. One day, when they had gone to this friend's house, after dinner and drinks, the friend proposed in a casual way to Arun that it would be a good idea for them to swap

Yes Darling, No Darling, Hello Darling

wives in the bedroom. Arun laughed at the proposal, not in dismissal but as in 'What a good idea'. Fortunately for Kiran, the friend's wife objected and the idea was dropped.

It also came out that amongst his friends, Arun was the life of the party, warmly greeted and feted. He would describe in detail the changes he had brought to the Club of which he had become President. Arun wore two different personae, one at home and the other outside. Everything Kiran did at home came under severe criticism and everything the hostesses at their parties did, received fulsome praise.

Kiran would confide in one of her close friends all that was going on in her life, and each time the friend advised her to put an end to this treatment by giving Arun an ultimatum that she would walk out of the marriage to end her misery. Her friend even suggested reporting the matter to the police; and certainly not taking any more nonsense. Kiran would sometimes agree with her friend but could never pick up the courage to make the move. A week later, there would be another phone call to her friend to narrate the slap she had received because the porridge was too cold. Why did she bring it to the table when he was still getting ready? Kiran was living the life of a victim, day after day, month after month, and year after year. Over the years, Kiran, who had come to her husband's home as a young and beautiful bride, turned into a fat and frumpy woman. Who cared about her looks anyway?

If my readers think that to bear such gross treatment for thirty years and do nothing about it is too hard to believe, let me remind you that Kiran is not the lone victim living in an abusive marriage. There are many more Kirans than we believe. But in India, the economic and social dependence of the wife on her husband; the lack of parental support in case the wife wants to make an issue of it; and the very male oriented society we live in, make it almost impossible for the Kirans of the world to do anything to change their fate.

Yes Darling, No Darling, Hello Darling

Listening to he during the following the sessions to understand the context of her marriage, I came to the conclusion that it would take a long time to help her get back on her feet. Thirty years is a long period over which both the personality and will to act, get destroyed. Therefore it could take her years to move from her current position to the one she desired to be in. I decided to use what I sometimes describe as 'changing the script' approach to counselling. This method will become clear as we proceed.

I told Kiran it was time to move into the 'payback' phase and explained by saying: "When Arun behaves in an abusive manner and you accept it, as you have been doing for all these years, he is writing the script of your life and you are acting strictly as per his script… 'I will abuse. She will take it. I will cut her down to size in the presence of the children and she will meekly submit. I will call her a no good woman in the presence of my brothers and she will lump it.' I told Kiran the time had come for her to reverse the roles and become the scriptwriter and let Arun play the role according to her script. Initially, the thought shocked her.

I knew I was taking a risk with this approach but risk-taking becomes necessary to deal with a person who has lived in an abusive marriage for so many years. One could wait for five years to see a situation like this change. I had decided to go with my own counselling and life experiences. My instincts told me such husbands are generally big bullies who kow-tow to their bosses at work and hate themselves for it; they regain their self-esteem by cutting others down to size. I have yet to meet a self-assured, self-confident person who respects himself, yet treats his wife or others badly. In my opinion, Arun fell into the category of people who hated themselves for being persons of low worth but put on a façade of being bullies to get along in life.

I told Kiran that from that day on, whenever she was given a mouthful, whatever the context, at home or outside, at the dining table or drawing rooml, in the bedroom or outside, she was to DISENGAGE. By which

Yes Darling, No Darling, Hello Darling

I meant moving out quietly with grace, the posture giving Arun the clear message that 'I, Kiran, have no time to waste on you, Arun'. "Position yourself in a manner to come across as a person who belongs to a superior league and will not waste time on coarse behaviour." I said to her. "Act like a queen, and surprise Arun. He won't know how to react because the only response that is wired in his brain is that you will meekly submit."

Getting her to fully understand how to follow the 'write your script' approach was quite a task but that was understandable. Imagine a wife who has been reduced to the position of a doormat by her husband, trying to take such a position! Just as Arun's neural circuits were wired to command and control, her circuits were wired to obey and submit. She finally agreed to follow my suggestions but had one or two doubts. Her first question was: If she disobeyed and he shouted, what should be her response? I told her to stand at a place where her husband's shouting could be heard by the neighbours and they could witness his behaviour. The study of psychology tells us that those who have built their reputations – sometimes I give it the label of brand equity – on falsehoods, like Arun had done, feel shamefaced to be caught with their pants down. "What if he keeps quiet but later slaps me when I am alone?" she then asked. I told her to shout for the children and slap back even harder. "Shock him!" I kept repeating. I also told her to call me if things got out of hand, and to leave the rest to me.

There was no call for two days and when I met her again she told me she had followed my advice. Arun had been shocked indeed. All he could do was push her out of the bedroom. She had slept in the guest room. The next morning, Arun had started the day by telling her never to dare do it again if she knew what was good for her. She had kept her counsel. It was the first of the month – the day she usually got the money for household expenses – but Arun walked out of the house without giving her any, leaving behind, as usual, his wish list for dinner. Kiran wanted to know what she should do next.

Yes Darling, No Darling, Hello Darling

Having achieved some success with this approach, I told her to take the no-money-no-dinner, approach. She agreed to try this new tack.

When Arun returned and asked his son where his mother was, he was told she had gone out for a stroll around the colony and that there was no dinner prepared, 'because mom said you had forgotten to give her the money for rations'. Arun was livid and began shouting at her even in her absence. Their son took exception to his father's behaviour but received a slap in return. The son went up to his room, packed his backpack and got ready to leave home. When Arun asked him where he was headed, he said he was going to spend the night with a friend and walked out, banging the door. Now Arun had another rebellion at home. When Kiran got back, Arun was on the phone ordering home delivery from a nearby restaurant. Kiran tiptoed to the guest room, locked herself in and switched on the TV very loud. Arun was left huffing and puffing, not knowing how to handle this totally new scenario which he was not prepared for. So he did what he was good at and drank himself silly, abusing Kiran loudly before turning in. Kiran took her own time to come out. She ate in the safety of her room and went to sleep. She did not emerge until Arun had left for work. Arun also got the news that his son had extended his stay with his friend for the long weekend ahead.

Kiran is still in counselling with me. The breakthrough achieved in her life is that she is now living in a disengaged marriage and has nothing to do with Arun except that they live under the same roof and run their lives on parallel tracks. She goes to the club to play cards with her friends, parties with them, and has her childrens' support. Arun goes to the factory and spends lonely evenings. After having lived the yes darling-no darling-hello darling façade, it is difficult for him to admit to others that his marriage has broken into pieces. They live in disengaged engagement with each other.

I mentioned 'changing the script' approach. Let us reflect on this. Ask yourself, is the agenda of your life being set by someone else? Is the

Yes Darling, No Darling, Hello Darling

script of your life being written by someone else – your spouse, your friends or family? Also ask whether you sometimes dance to the tune selected and played by someone else? If, on reflection, you conclude your answer is in the affirmative, this may be the time to wake up to reality and avoid landing yourself in a situation akin to Kiran's.

This insight about dancing to others' tunes came to me at a workshop I attended (the same workshop mentioned in the previous chapter). The rule about punctuality was strictly enforced at the workshop. We were often reminded about it and those who came late were given a dressing down in public. But all this had no effect on one participant. He was perpetually late – except on the last day. The workshop leader was surprised to see the chronic latecomer sitting in his assigned chair and asked him how come he was on time.

The man went on the offensive, saying he had had enough of the leader's haranguing and did not want to hear it repeated. So he had missed his breakfast, driven fast, and gone past red lights to reach the session on time. When he finished his story, the leader's response was loud and clear, not only for him but for all of us: "So you missed your breakfast, right?" The man nodded. "You drove recklessly, right?" Another nod. "You broke the traffic rules, right?" The man got irritated and said, "Yes, yes, yes!" There was a pause, followed by the leader's punch line directed at us all: "For your colleague here, I was the puppeteer and he was the puppet. I pulled one string and he missed his breakfast. I pulled another string and he drove recklessly. Yet another string pulled and shooting a red light resulted. Choose to be a puppet if you wish to be." The message was hard to miss.

Plainly speaking, you may have given the power of your life to someone else. Over time, it can happen that you accept and act on others' bidding and become something of a doormat over which all and sundry walk. What I am saying is not an exaggeration but the reality of many lives. If that be your case, then write down the names of those whose wishes and fancies you may have surrendered to and take back from them the

Yes Darling, No Darling, Hello Darling

power of your life into your own hands. Declare to yourself: I will no longer accept a lose-win relationship in which I am the loser and the other is the winner. Initially, there will be a lot of resistance from those who have enjoyed power over you, but if you are consistent in your behaviour, they will get the message. There will still be some who will want to call the shots. The best you can do is to disengage from such people – and that includes those in your immediate family – because no one has the right to degrade you as a human being. Walk with your head high, not from arrogance but self-esteem and self-respect. Period.

Let us examine a few other aspects about marital relationships and how some marriages are examples of harmony while others reflect pain and discord. The first category is one in which each partner provides the other space to grow; to follow their own interests and pursuits; have their own circle of friends; decide what they choose to read. The couple live as friends. The platform is 'I love you and therefore I need you', and not 'I need you, therefore I love you'. The next thing that disturbs the harmony of marital music is expectations, which are often not even expressed. 'She should know I like my tea very hot' etc. A host of expectations is a big destroyer of marriages. The third aspect, very relevant in India, is the sense of ownership of an object called the spouse. 'How dare she do this without my permission?' or 'This is not how a husband behaves'.

Should, should and more shoulds are the sources of disease in married life. I would even go as far to say the word 'should' needs to be excluded from the dictionary. There is something slavish about it. 'I should do this because my husband wants it.' 'I should do so otherwise what will people say?' The word 'could' gives us options, but 'should' has the flavour of control and snatches away freedom. I end with two statements made by Eleanor Roosevelt, about self-respect: 'No one can take away your self-respect without your consent' and 'I know that we will be the sufferers if we let great wrongs occur without exerting ourselves to correct them.'

Yes Darling, No Darling, Hello Darling

GURUSPEAK ON ABUSIVE MARRIAGES

The first thing we need to realise is that abusive marriages are much more common than we would like to believe. In most cases, the victims are not even clear as to what remedial steps they ought to take. Many victims continue to live in abusive marriages because their *roti, kapda* and *makaan* (subsistence) depend on their husbands. They live in hope that, with the passage of time, the abuse will diminish or disappear. But the results are exactly the opposite. The marriage lives on hope.

If I was to think of one major reason for the perpetuation of abuses, it would be the extremely low self-esteem of the abused person. Remember Kiran's case? It took her thirty long years before she dared to step out and speak. Superimposed on this issue are stupid, unfounded, drilled-in-the-head beliefs that marriages are made in heaven, so you have to accept living in marital hell all one's life. Then there is the grossly misunderstood religious belief that husbands are ten steps higher in the hierarchal ladder than wives. There is a book by a Muslim cleric which has a chapter on why husbands should beat their wives; the use of sticks and slaps is permitted. I leave it to your judgement.

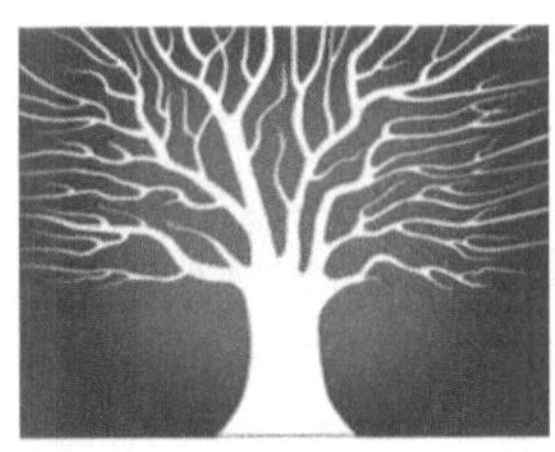

Beauty lies in the eye of the beer holder. ~ Anonymous

Much against my wishes, I had to locate to Delhi for a year for professional reasons. I continued with my counselling practice because I believed that, like any skill, you need to stay in practice. It takes a long time to acquire a skill but is easy to lose. The case narrated below happened during my tenure in Delhi.

The first bridal kiss she received from her now late husband, almost thirty years ago, was laced with alcohol. The emotional trauma of her life started that night. She lived with it for thirty years because she did not have the courage to see a counsellor, and she came to me only when pushed by the older of her two sons. Thirty years of wasted life, thirty years of emotional trauma and deep scars, and thirty years of living in an abusive marriage and a subservient life dictated by her late husband's family – and that too, when she had an independent source of income – because her religious teachings almost forbade her to seek help. 'Pray, yes, read the scriptures, yes, but no going to a counsellor' was the mindset she had acquired over time.

Wamil was an educated woman who drew attention whenever she entered a room. She must have been a beauty in her day. She reminded me of an Urdu poem: *Khandar bata rahe hain, Imarat azeem thi* (the relics are telling us that the building was beautiful). When she came to see me, she told me her immediate issue, which was the position her family had taken vis-à-vis herself. It went like this: 'Now that you are a widow and your sons are working away from the city, you have all the time to spend nights with our mother who is not well and look after her for most of the day too.' Wamil submitted. 'Now that you are a widow you have all the

From Victim To Victor

time at your disposal to look after our kids while we go on holiday.' 'Now that you are a widow and have time, cook a delicious Chinese meal for the family.' These examples represented what her life was all about. She gave me so many examples of the non-negotiable orders she received from her brothers and their wives; her sisters and their husbands. To me, the message the family was giving her was this: Now that you are a widow, you are a doormat and we can walk all over you.

In counselling, we generally do not classify our cases as the most successful or unsuccessful because we know that comparisons between humans get you anywhere. However, if I were to make an exception, I would classify this as the most successful case. Thirty years of tyranny was resolved in three months. But let me begin from the beginning.

Wamil was married to a confirmed alcoholic and his family knew it. But then, in India, marriage is often used to pass the buck because it is getting too much for us or we truly believe marriage will dissolve depression, addictions, compulsive disorders, irresponsible attitudes and the like. We never seem to learn that instead of one family bearing the brunt of the issue, there will be two living in misery. But we continue to believe, if marriage does not solve the problem, the arrival of children will – as though sex opens new neural circuits of wisdom and obliterates the old destructive ones.

It did not take an educated Wamil long to realise her husband was a confirmed alcoholic. Often, he would start the day with the bottle. She tried everything a person unfamiliar with the subject of alcoholism could do, but nothing worked. Hiding the bottles only added to her husband's fury. Most of us do not realise that alcoholics often take a vow in the morning that they will never ever touch the bottle but soon succumb to the habit and find ways and means of satisfying their addiction. Wamil's life was a misery. She would wait until her husband arrived late at night and open the door only to be dragged out, slapped and locked out. Ashamed, she did not mention her travails even to her friends. As far as her husband's family was concerned, it was no longer

From Victim To Victor

their business. It was not much different with her own family either. It was her *kismet*, her fate.

Wamil's two sons were the only source of happiness and in these difficult circumstances; she did all she could to bring them up with the love they should have received from both parents. She did not accept the invitations from close family and friends for one reason – she did not want to let down her husband in their eyes. Her social life came to a grinding halt. Soon she was left to herself. Some people labelled her a snooty woman. Wamil began seeing herself as a person of no worth and her self-esteem went crashing down to the ground.

This is an abridged version of her terrible life. But in one area she came out a big-ticket winner. Her sons grew up to be successful professionals. Recognising that the foundations of what they had achieved had been laid by their mother, they both did everything to pay back their debt of gratitude. As I mentioned earlier, the elder son, who was in touch with the reality of today's world, literally pushed her along the path to counselling.

I knew that in this case normal counselling approaches would take years to bring Wamil anywhere close to recovering her self-worth. She had too many scars to heal and needed to be supported by the counsellor's direction. I decided to abandon the non-directive way of counselling for a directive one. This helps in cases where the counselee comes to us in a battered state, such as Wamil's. The counsellor takes charge when he thinks it is worth taking the risk. It also helps when a counselee sees the counsellor as a role model. Intuition, in such cases, is a big help. What is your inner voice telling you? What is your gut feeling telling you? Some would argue against this stance. However, I believe that with human beings, we cannot use the one-shoe-fits-all approach. I am a strong believer in following intuitive messages, even if logic says otherwise. In three different business situations in the past, I had settled for what looked like good decisions and shut off my inner voice. On all three occasions my fingers got burnt.

From Victim To Victor

I instantly decided to use the 'fake-it-till-you-make-it' approach and fortunately, Wamil agreed to follow my directions implicitly. My gut feeling and life's experience told me she was dealing with bullies who would blink. We shook hands on the decision. I told her to go home instead of going to her mother's house as planned. She responded that her mother would report this to her elder brother, who would ring up and demolish her. My reply was that the time was long overdue for her to demolish her family; they deserved the same treatment they had meted out to her. I advised her not to take any calls from those from whom she expected a backlash and to be consistent in that approach.

Fortunately, Wamil stuck by it. She refused to see those who wanted to call on her to pressurize her. It happened sooner than I had expected; the family hired two nurses to take care of the mother and began sharing some of the duties Wamil had been performing single-handedly. They had no option but to accept the new situation. In about six weeks, they began treating her as an equal. That made her feel good about herself.

In the next few sessions, I explained to Wamil that all her life she had lived in a state of co-dependency and now she had finally moved on to be independent of the family. But that was not enough, because it was time for her to move to the beautiful stage of interdependency. That meant, drawing up a list of friends who were dear to her; inviting them over and relating with them; going out with them and socializing; and living the life that was her basic right. Wamil said every step I asked her to take was fully supported by her son, who would often say, "Mum, this is what I have been telling you all the while but you would not listen."

In the next session, she asked me why I did not suggest meeting her friends before this. I explained that it was only when she had tasted independence that she would find the courage to move into an interdependence mode. Things are working beautifully for her and she keeps in touch, not to seek help but to share her happiness. In such cases, counsellors have to remind themselves not to let the success stories go to their heads but say instead: 'I am blessed I have not had to go through such torrid experiences as those who come to me have gone through.' Never forget that today a counsellor can be in a state of congruence but tomorrow is another day.

What is being in a congruent state? Those who have an elementary knowledge of geometry will know what an equilateral triangle is – a triangle where all sides are equal. With human beings, congruence means being in a similar state of equilibrium – that the mind, heart and physique are in sync and all three are aligned to the issue in front of us. Our body language and words are in a state of harmony and we are there in the present. We are happy with what we are. We are not suffering from 'shoulds' such as, 'I should have done that' or 'I should be doing that' (a state in which we are in conflict). Congruence is a happy state in which we are comfortable with ourselves and there are minimal internal conflicts. Incongruence is exactly the opposite, with conflicts in the mind: 'Should I do this or that?' We are troubled and our emotions exceed what we should be facing given the circumstances. In a counselling room, this may mean the counsellor is in a relatively congruent state but not the counselee. Lest it be misunderstood that counsellors should be in congruence all the time – that is certainly not possible and would be asking for *nirvana* or a mystical state. The idea is that the counsellor should be in a here-and-now state in the counselling room; able to focus on the client's thoughts and feelings.

In many cases, I have observed that when a minor infraction is imposed on a client, he says to himself: 'I won't allow it the next time'. But having accepted it once, the person succumbs again, saying; 'I will put my foot down the next time'. As the demands pile up, the hurdle gradually gets higher and higher, and climbing over it becomes too difficult. Sooner rather than later the person loses his self-esteem and submitting to someone else's will becomes a habit. We cannot forget that no one – but no one – has the right to transgress the boundaries of our self-respect.

DEALING WITH ALCOHOLICS AND THEIR FAMILIES

Although counsellors are trained to deal with many lifestyle issues, handling drug and alcohol abuse does not come easy to most of us. On a personal level, I refer such cases to organisations dedicated to working in this domain, such as Alcohol Anonymous (AA) or drug de-addiction centres. But as counsellors we do meet those who have someone very close in the family who is substance dependent.

It is thus important to be familiar with issues related to such social problems. The person who comes to us may be the spouse or someone so closely related to the drug addict/alcoholic, that the addict is bound to cast a shadow on the client's life. First, we need to be constantly aware that dependence becomes a habit that is not easy to break and that the victim of substance/alcohol abuse is suffering as much, if not more, than the people close to him. Never, never take a judgmental position about the victim. I say this with all the unambiguous emphasis at my command since I have often heard comments like: 'That idiot has hit the bottle again. It serves him right that all his friends have ditched him' or 'He is back in the de- addiction centre'. Therefore, as we counsel and empathise with those who come to us, we also need to have a better understanding about the issues that confront them.

In many cases, the issue of alcoholism lies in the genes of the person. Depression and anxiety can also lead to addiction. Or it may be an abusive marriage that leads to it. Sometimes a breakdown in family relationships makes a person hide behind the bottle or drugs. Also, people do not seek help in many cases because of the embarrassment it brings to them and their families. And we also see cases where those who are closely related, begin to feel guilty for two reasons: one – could they have been the cause of the problem? And two – could they be doing more than they have been doing, to alleviate the victim's pain? As counsellors, we have to help to remove this guilt syndrome.

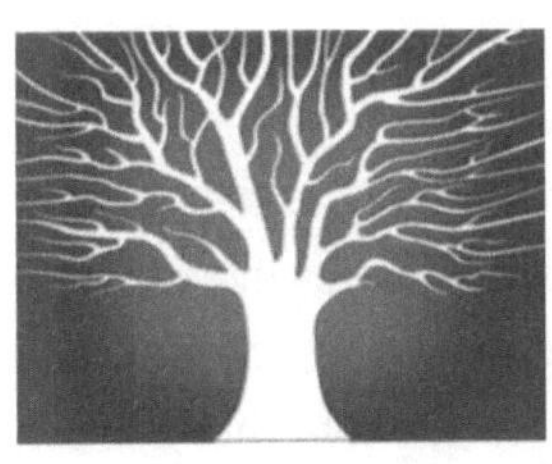

Be who you are and say what you feel because those who mind don't matter and those who matter don't mind. ~ Dr Seuss

To hell with others – this four-word sentence is a curse. My inner response to this has always been: If we cannot look after ourselves, not in a selfish but in a self-esteeming way; and spend time speculating what other people will say or do instead, we are sure to tie ourselves in veritable knots of perpetual pain. In a world of billions, how many are we going to satisfy?

This is just what Prakash and his family were trying to do for the last fifteen years, at the cost of their daughter's happiness and their grandson's future – "to save face" (to use an Indian idiom). Prakash's daughter, Jyoti, was nineteen when, based on her hard work, she gained admission to a college in the US. Jyoti, who had shown maturity well beyond her age, was denied permission to go abroad by her family, for fear that she was too young to be left alone in a foreign country. Jyoti lost the scholarship and with it her dream of studying further.

Jyoti's family, though economically well-to-do, were bound by tradition. They did what many such families do – rush to tie the proverbial knot for their daughter through an arranged marriage. In many arranged marriages the girl particularly has no say in the matter. In Jyoti's case, every decision was taken by the parents. When all the details had been finalised, she was asked what she thought of the boy and his family. Jyoti knew it was just a formality being gone through to evade any responsibility if things did not work out in the future. Then the parents could fall back on it and say, '*Beti*, we asked what you felt about the match and you did not say anything'.

What will People Say?

So Jyoti married Suresh, a software engineer. In less than a week, Jyoti found something strange about Suresh's behaviour. She heard him talking to himself and often saw him standing in front of the mirror, having a conversation with his reflection. She found this very strange but kept her counsel. When this behaviour began to disturb her, she talked it over with her parents, who advised her to see whether Suresh was taking any medicines. Jyoti kept a watchful eye and discovered that her mother-in-law would add a few drops of medicine with a dropper into Suresh's coffee every morning. When Jyoti reported this to her parents, she was asked to note down the name of the medicine Suresh was being given.

Jyoti's father then consulted a psychiatrist, to be told that the medicine was usually prescribed to those suffering from mental illness. The doctor said it was difficult to make a clear assessment without meeting the young man, but he suspected Suresh could be suffering from schizophrenia; he explained what the disease was. Jyoti's father was extremely disturbed and asked her to see if she could lay her hands on the prescription and the name of the doctor who had started the process of medication. Jyoti ferreted out the information and concluded Suresh had been visiting a well-known psychiatrist in Delhi. Prakash then set up a meeting with the doctor to get a confirmation that Suresh was indeed schizophrenic. The doctor confirmed the diagnosis and said Suresh would have to be kept on medication for as long as the doctor felt it was necessary.

A few words on schizophrenia would be in order here. It is a psychotic disease that distorts the reality of a person and leads to faulty thinking and withdrawal from social contact. It literally disintegrates the process of thinking and makes one emotionally dysfunctional. A side effect can be depression; I have known patients who entirely lose touch with reality. One such patient would come to me for counselling because he needed to talk to someone. But he would threaten me saying if I did not do something fast to help him recover, he would report my poor performance to General Musharraf (then President of Pakistan).

What will People Say?

In Suresh's case, the disease was reflected in the very unconventional way he dressed and the grandiose statements he made. Even more noticeable, while most software engineers carry their laptops in a bag, Suresh used a big box, in which he would carry not just the laptop but CDs with all his software; he also saved his data and lectures of Osho, as well as music on pen drives. In fact, his entire home office went along with him. It was just a matter of time before he was fired. The family blamed Jyoti for all the ills her husband faced.

When Jyoti came to see me, enough mess had already been created in her life because of the 'what will people say' policy followed by her parents: 'Stick with Suresh, otherwise what will people say?' 'Don't say a word to anyone, including your friends, otherwise what will people say?' 'Look after Suresh, he is your husband, otherwise what will people say?' The result was that instead of resolving Jyoti's issues, the situation was compounded when she got pregnant. Caught between her parents' dictates and her in-laws' accusations, Jyoti felt helpless. Abortion was out of the question because she was too far gone to have that option. In any case, her parents told her, her life would be lovely once the bundle of joy arrived on the scene. As a counsellor I knew that the new arrival too, might suffer from the disease as it grew up since schizophrenia is known to pass, in some cases, from parent to offspring.

When I saw Jyoti the first time, she too had expressed this 'what will people say' mindset. It came out when she would go back to her parents to get away from the stressful environment at home. But she would not join her parents when they visited friends or attended events, worried what people would say when they knew she had been away from her husband for two months.

After two months of weekly visits to me, I asked Jyoti and her father what they felt they could change in the behaviour of Suresh and his mother? The reply was that they had no control over them – one was mentally sick and the other had adopted an aggressive posture and made Jyoti and her parents responsible for Suresh's condition. I used an analogy I often apply to bring home the point – if one were to continue to travel on the same track, one would visit the same station one had been visiting in the past. I suggested they change tracks in order to get to a different destination. They insisted I choose the track for them. But it is not for the counsellor to decide if the issue can be resolved by the caretakers – in this case, the parents. Although there is a strong temptation to do so, let such choices be made by the counselee or those looking after the person. The maximum a counsellor may do, to my mind, is add to the menu of choices made by the counselee.

Both Jyoti and her father fell back into the 'what will people say' mindset and I had to regretfully terminate counselling. There is no point to the counselling process if no progress is taking place. Many new counsellors see termination of counselling in these conditions as personal failures. But counselling is a joint venture between the counsellor and counselees and if any in this joint venture cannot add further value to the process, there is no point labouring over it. Some other recourse has to be found.

To my surprise, Prakash rang me to set up another appointment, and after a couple of sessions with me and the doctors about Suresh's chances of recovery, he finally concluded they should move the court for divorce. Jyoti filed the case only to face the wrath of Suresh's aggressive mother, who believed that the source of all the problems were, in fact, Jyoti and her parents. In this narrative, you will observe there has been no mention of Suresh's father. Whenever the subject of Suresh's condition came up, he would be missing. He would go up to the roof of the house or step out to attend to some urgent work. Maybe he knew the truth – only he can tell. But the sad part is that while all this was going on, Jyoti and her family continued to harp on the cursed sentence: What will people say? Jyoti's twelve-year-old son got sadly stuck in the mire and developed a faraway look and became a loner.

What will People Say?

If we spend our time and energies on other people's reactions, let this case be the reminder that running our lives on *what will people say*, is a zero sum game.

POSTSCRIPT

I happened to meet Jyoti a couple of years later and learned that, on the advice of her parents and relatives, she had withdrawn the divorce case. She told me that since her brother was then of a marriageable age, 'everyone' felt the court case would be a slur on the family and the chances of his finding the right bride would suffer. She mentioned she had taken over the duty of adding the medicines to Suresh's coffee – a task previously performed by his mother. She also told me she and her son were both under treatment for depression. A heavy price for keeping others happy.

At the beginning of this chapter, I quoted Dr Seuss. I invite you to revisit the quote and see if it makes better sense now.

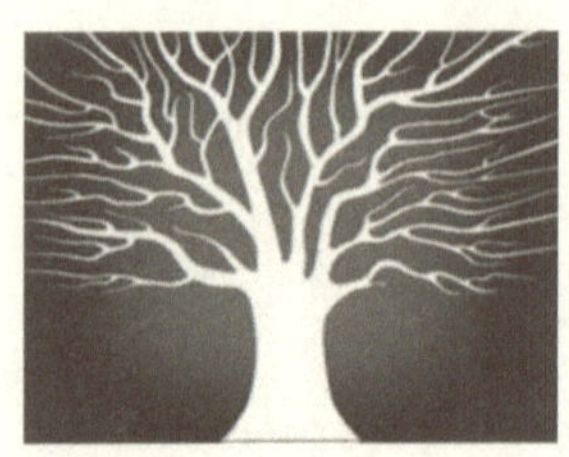

Why would you have your cake and not eat it? Anonymous

Varsha came to see me through the reference of a friend of mine who lived in the same apartment complex she did. After the initial introductions, Varsha got to the point straight away – she wanted counselling because she could not bear her life anymore. In most cases, as you too will have noticed, clients have difficulty in stating the issue they have come to resolve. There are doubts upon doubts. 'Do I really want counselling?' 'Will it help?' 'Am I wasting my time?' 'What if my friends come to know?' I have known cases where clients have said: 'I went past your counselling centre six months ago but did not have the courage to come in and seek help. I came back last month but retraced my steps. Three days ago, I almost entered the room but stepped back. Today, I decided, for whatever its worth, to go in and seek help.' Varsha did not seem to have any such doubts.

Twenty-four-year-old Varsha, an architect by training, came to see me one day. She had excelled professionally at a young age. She had even gone to England to do a diploma in landscaping after her degree in architecture. She found a job in a small firm run by an entrepreneur architect, Gautam, who was twelve years her senior. The firm had no shortage of assignments and the two of them, with support staff, worked mostly with repeat customers. Spending 8-10 hours together in the office and travelling to meet clients on-site, led to intimacy which resulted in going to Gautam's home after work, enjoying the evening with him over wine, followed by quick sex, and then getting home by dinner time. The story of being overworked and so returning late, carried on for over a year.

Having his Cake and Eating it Too

She noticed that when she was relatively free on weekends, Gautam would leave early without even telling her. When this carried on for some weeks, she mentioned it to one of the draughtsman and was told that on Saturdays, Gautam's separated wife visited him from Mysore to take care of the dogs she loved so much. When Varsha confronted Gautam with this, he threw a tantrum and said he was the victim of circumstances. His wife would not discuss divorce. He was helpless. He asked that they continue the love affair. When she refused, he went mad, shouted at her and called her a letdown, so Varsha succumbed and their physical relationship carried on for months, only because she did not pick up the courage to put a stop to it. And that was why she was seeking help.

I complimented Varsha on her decision and asked her what options she saw before her. She said she had even resigned in order to move out but Gautam had cried and told her it was she who had done so much to build the business and she could not leave and create a vacuum. He called her a selfish person and Varsha had fallen into line. After some time, she cursed her own weakness. This pattern was repeated many times.

After that first session, I began to reflect on Varsha's issue, to see what direction it could be headed. Reflection, on the part of the counsellor, is very important to seek clarity on the future course of action. Her behaviour indicated a strong dependency on her male partner, otherwise why she would she surrender herself in bed just because he threw tantrums?

I started the second session by asking Varsha to narrate her growing years, starting from the time she remembered. Regression into childhood gives the therapist a whole lot of clues on the personality fix of the person. And this is what Varsha had to tell me. Her father was a semi-educated person in the construction business. He had the resources to send her and her two siblings to good schools and provide them with a comfortable life. Her mother was an educationist

Having his Cake and Eating it Too

who ran a school. There was little communication between her parents as they had no common ground. Her father would come home late and be disrespectful to his wife. So far as the children were concerned, there was no communication with their father except for angry words when he disapproved of their behaviour. Although the family lived in the same house, each was left to manage their own life. Varsha confessed that there was no bonding in the family, no going out together. They were like separate pillars of the same house. She found it frustrating to hear her friends talk about family picnics and weekend outings.

What has been narrated here in gist, gave me the tentative clue that Varsha's excessive dependency on Gautam could be on account of her rootless upbringing. Could it be that Gautam had become the anchor she badly needed? In the next session, guided by my own intuition, I decided to try a totally different approach. It often works well but the couusellor has to be ready to backtrack when it fails. I asked Varsha that given the mess she was in, what options did she have to move forward? She got upset and complained that was precisely the reason she had come for counselling, to seek advice.

"But that is your problem. And you must have some solution for solving your own problem." The more she protested, the more I persisted. When she found that I continued to put the ball in her court, she said she could end the relationship and stop going to work. We discussed that option but she wanted to have more sessions and see if she could get Gautam to come along with her. We ended our session on that note and fixed the date for the next session.

Gautam and Varsha turned up together. I saw Varsha first and she said that she felt she did not have the courage to tell Gautam by herself that she wanted to end the relationship. She felt more secure saying this to Gautam in my presence. When asked how she would put it across to him, her responses were very feeble and she had to rehearse her statements over and over again to put some energy into her vocal chords. I then met Gautam, who made a big case of how he could not live without Varsha. He was so dependent on her during work and after work. When asked about the status of his marriage, he had this to say: "I can't help it if the bloody woman won't get out of my life. I am helpless. But it should not have any effect on my relationship with Varsha because she comes to visit me only on weekends." He made a great case for continuing his relationship with Varsha.

I called Varsha in at that stage and told her, in summary, Gautam's views. She stood up and said boldly and clearly that she was quitting both the job and the relationship. Gautam went berserk and started ranting. He even said that I had tricked her into making the decision. I kept calm. When Gautam found that nothing was working for him, he stormed out of the room. I had many more sessions with Varsha to bring back her self-esteem. The more we talked about her past, the more it became clear that she was still hurting from the scars of early childhood, having been brought up in a dysfunctional family. I remember reading somewhere and it has been reinforced in my counselling, that the family is an organization, just like a company. The company that places emphasis 'quality first' as their philosophy, produces quality products. Profits are the result of that philosophy. The same applies to families. Those that nurture children, produce wholesome, confident, self-esteemed grown-ups. And finally, Varsha too, flew out of her cage of insecurity and dependency.

GURUSPEAK: DEPENDENCY

It is said that the children who grow up with alcoholic parents attract alcoholic partners in later life. In many cases, children who grow up in dysfunctional families like Varsha's, become passive personalities and look for anchors to support their lives; they often lean on someone similar from their early childhood. Varsha's father was abusive, so was Gautam. Such people tend to take over the responsibility that belongs to others. They cannot stand the loss of a relationship, however imbalanced the equation.

Having his Cake and Eating it Too

Varsha was willing to work hard at office and after office, even when she knew Gautam was not going to divorce his wife. Dependent people allow others to have their cake and eat it too. Their relationships becomes traps they cannot escape from. Why does that happen? Clearly, because of the lack of love in early childhood, they remain insecure as adults. Their constant concern is that if they free themselves of the relationship, they would be left high and dry. Being unsure of themselves, they tolerate abuse even if they are let down. This type of dependency does not build lasting relationships. Unless they are helped, through counselling, and made to feel they are persons of worth, they languish in poor relationships. They stay dependent children even in adulthood. One thing is certain –dependency destroys the personality of the dependent.

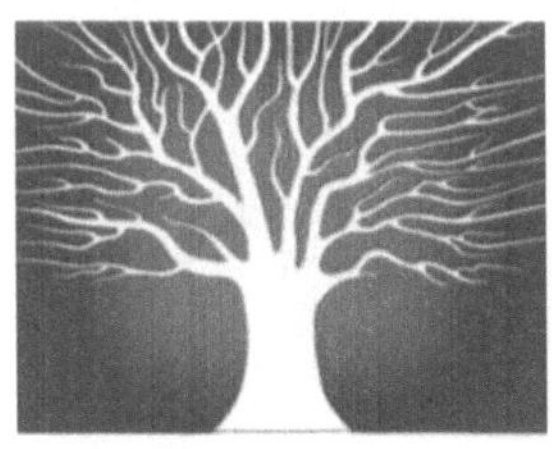

There was a time when weekly columns were written by experienced counsellors in the print media, on issues dealing with emotional health. Now, the media does not find space for counselling issues as they are too preoccupied with the physical aspects of our lives. I believe they are short-changing their readers thereby. Physical and mental health do not rest on two separate pillars, disconnected from each other. Physical and mental health are symbiotic, integrated and connected. Many depressed people find remedy in resorting to physical exercise and gain by it.

In my free time, I write short pieces on emotional health issues. It is my sincere hope that these articles will provide some insights into living the life all of us are entitled to. If we do not live wholesome and positive lives ourselves, there is not much chance of our living interdependent lives with others. That is my unshakeable belief.

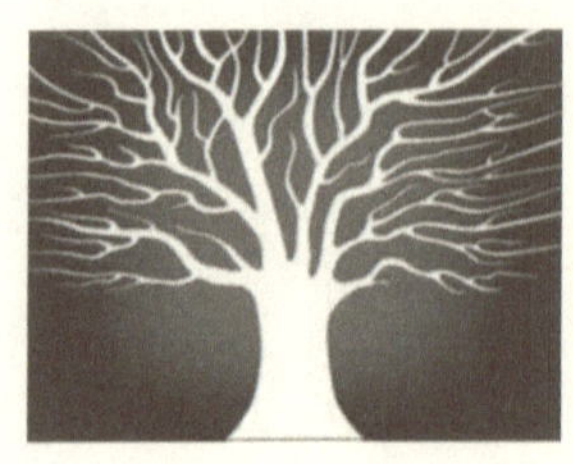

It is my view, any attempt at providing counselling services remains incomplete if confined only to the physical, mental and emotional domains, and does not, at the appropriate time, move into the realm of spirituality. This opinion may be at variance with that held by counsellors who possess a scientific temper, but before the argument gets too loud, let me call Dr Carl Jung to my defence. He says: *There has not been one (patient) whose problem in the last resort was not that of finding a religious outlook on life. It is safe to say every one of them fell ill because he had lost that which the living religions of every age have given their followers, and none of them has really healed who did not regain his religious outlook.* Here we can read 'spiritual' for religious. It will be easier to understand the concept of spirituality if we see it within a context. Take the example of marital counselling. The conventional approach takes us as far as clarifying and exchanging expectations of the spouses. Much time is spent on this effort, as in facilitating the couple's understanding of each other's background and biases.

But I personally believe that the stage arrives in the process of counselling, when we must question the very basis of having expectations at all. The couple can be made to understand that the source of their problem is clinging to expectations. If, having realized this, the partners are able to say to each other: 'I free you to be yourself, to think your thoughts, to indulge your tastes, follow your inclinations, and behave in any way you decide. I release you from all expectations. I accept you the way you are,' now would that not be liberating? Who has bestowed on us the right to expect anything from another? This is a good question to ask oneself.

Spirituality & Counselling: An Alternative View

Those who come for counselling are unhappy people. The source of unhappiness is different in each case. Personally, I would like to see counselling philosophy include Buddha's teachings, which tell us that the source of all unhappiness is either our craving for something or our aversion to something. If we meditate on this deeply, we find this to be true. It is either our craving to dominate in a relationship or aversion to being dominated, which is the source of our unhappiness. Exchanging expectations between spouses is a temporary solution because expectations change. Dropping them leads to healing.

I hesitate to mention the word *karma* lest it be perceived as a Hindu bias, but what else is cause and effect if not *karma*? Saying that our destiny depends upon our *karma* is the same thing as saying the effect depends on the cause. In Buddhism, the principle of causality is accepted as a natural law, as the Dalai Lama has explained. In dealing with reality, we have to take that law into account. So, for instance, in the case of everyday experiences, if there are certain events we do not desire to happen, the best method is to ensure that the conditions which normally cause them, do not exist. This is also true with mental states and experiences. If we desire happiness, we must seek what gives rise to it; and if we wish to avoid suffering, then we must ensure the causes and conditions that give rise to suffering no longer exist. Good old *karma is* at work in mental conditions and therapy as well.

There are those who grapple with negative thoughts that limit their lives. One negative thought feeds another. A reason for negative thoughts troubling us is that we give them unnecessary importance and attention. Sometimes we do this in the process of counselling itself. The practice of meditation reveals to us that it is in the nature of thoughts to come and go, and the observation of thoughts in a non-judgmental way, dissolves them. Hence, should we not direct the counselled to various meditation techniques available to us? Meditation, which helps to dissolve negativity and enhance awareness, has caught the imagination of the Western world. Let us not forget it began here in India.

Spirituality & Counselling: An Alternative View

Then there is this spiritual law of impermanence. A friend of mine who went through a period of deep depression, shared with me that the most redeeming feature during this dark period, besides medicines and counselling, was his belief in the law of impermanence. Happy days do not last forever but by the same law, unhappy days also pass. Surely there is a lesson in this for us counsellors too, in dealing with cases of depression?

In cases of low self-esteem, attempts are often made at stroking the person and talking him out of it. I believe that acceptance of current reality is a much better approach to healing. From acceptance and surrender to current reality, we receive the positive energy to deal with any negative feelings. Dr M Scott Peck, in his book, *The Road Less Travelled,* is particularly harsh on his scientific colleagues. He says they suffer from a kind of tunnel vision: '…a psychologically self-imposed psychological set of blinders which prevents them from turning their attention to the realm of the spirit'. Because of this attitude, many scientists exclude from serious consideration, matters that are, or seem to be, intangible. In the chapter, The Miracle of Health, M. Scott Peck quotes the poem *Amazing Grace* by John Newton:

Amazing grace! How sweet the sound
That saved a wretch like me!
I once was lost but now am found
Was blind but now I see.
T'was grace that taught my heart to fear
And grace my fears relieved;
How precious did that grace appear
The hour I first believed!
Through many dangers, toils and snares
I have already come;
T'is grace hath brought me safe thus far
And grace will lead me home.
And when we've been there ten thousand years,
Bright shining as the sun
We'll have no less days to sing God's praise
Than when we first begun.

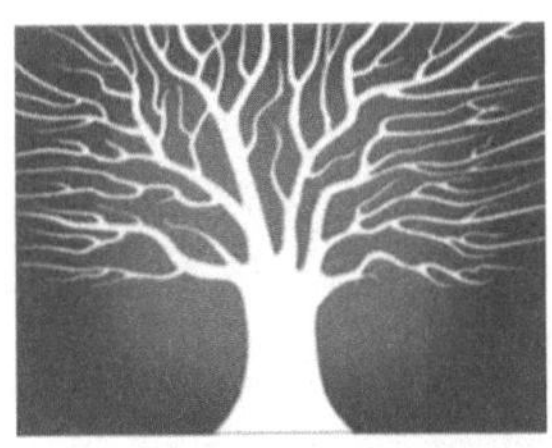

Are you living in an abusive marriage?

Recovering from abuse: Is it possible? It depends on you.

One look and I knew I was dealing with a broken spirit. Here was someone on the verge of a breakdown. One of my counselling colleagues nudged me to take her on for counselling. I gently guided the lady to a room and invited her to take a chair. She sat down hesitatingly, unsure of herself, frozen with fear. I mentioned my name and asked for hers. "Geeta," she whispered, but could not say another word. A light, empathetic touch on her knee and she broke down in uncontrollable sobs. It took her a long time to say: "I don't want to live. I just don't want to live with him." She kept repeating between sobs, "I can't stand it anymore. I just can't. It is too much."

In the course of the next few weekly sessions, the story of Geeta's miserable marriage unfolded. Her husband, a trader in tyres, would come home after work and for no reason, start abusing her, calling her a bitch, a good-for-nothing, who wasted her time while he worked hard. He would make statements like, "You bitch! If it was not for you, I would not have picked up this drinking habit." Geeta said that right from the first day of their marriage, she was not treated like a human being but as an object to be used in bed when it pleased him and then discarded.

I asked her how long she had been married and she replied: "Seventeen years". I said: "Seventeen years you have been in this relationship, and you have done nothing about it?" Geeta looked at me and sobbed, "What could I do, Uncle? Every time I brought the story of my miserable life to my parents' notice, they would either ask me to adjust or blame me for his behaviour."

It took almost five months of weekly counselling sessions for Geeta to recover her self-esteem, self-respect and regain her rightful position in the marriage. In this case, thankfully, the husband backed off, realizing that his abusive behaviour would not work anymore.

Geeta is representative of wives living in emotionally abusive relationships. Here are some of the clear signs of being in such a relationship:

- Your husband gets irritated for no reason. When you ask him why he is behaving in this way, he just denies it.
- When you want to talk to him about it, he says you are making too much of it.
- You begin to think there is something wrong with you.
- Whatever you say, he takes the opposite view just to annoy you.
- He threatens to stop giving you money or says something like: 'I can't live with you anymore', to blackmail you into submission.

Some husbands do not stop at verbal abuse but beat and bruise their wives, as in Geeta's case. She had ugly bruises on her arms; to hide her shame, she would tell her friends she had slipped in the bathroom, or wear clothes which hid the marks. Many women in India live lives of agony. This can be avoided by seeking counselling at a recognised counselling centre.

How does counselling help in such cases? The first thing a counsellor does is to listen, when no one else has. This intense sharing of one's misery with someone, through empathic listening, reduces the load the victim has been carrying on her shoulders for a long time. She begins to understand and accept that she is in no way the cause of her husband's anger and abuse – something she had begun to believe. The counsellor listens, shows compassion, and respects the person.

Are you living in an Abusive Marriage?

Over a period of time, when the person has been able to rid herself of guilt, shame and misery, she begins to see her position clearly and look at the options available. In my experience, when an abusive husband sees his wife will not take his nonsense anymore, he mends his ways. However, this is not always the case. Often the husband uses his economic strength to get his wife to remain in bondage.

The counselling process helps to make the wife more self-assured, to deal with her husband, and choose from a place of personal strength and not weakness. For example, she might choose to continue living in the marriage, disengage herself emotionally from her husband, training herself to take up a job; or she might decide that enough was enough and divorce was the best option. Whatever be the ultimate choice, she makes it herself, from personal power and strength, and not helplessness.

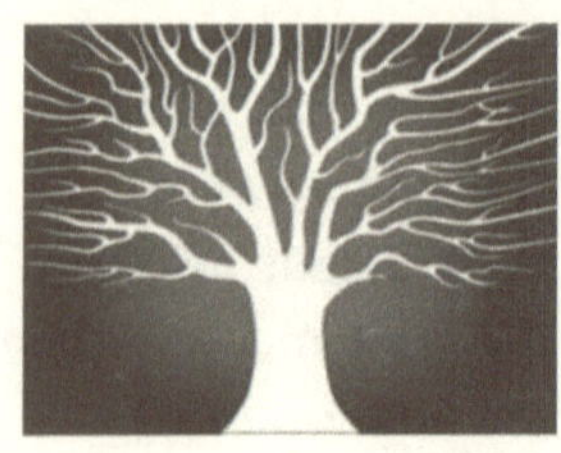

I do not know how many readers would agree with me that there are more unhappy marriages than happy ones. This chapter deals with some of the issues that make for happy marriages and those that do not. Let's start with an example. I have a friend who hates dancing, but his wife loves it. He is fond of attending public speaking classes and spends a lot of energy training himself as a speaker; but his wife hates the very thought of speaking in public. The ingredients of an unhappy marriage are present here. However, they are happy together. The reason: each provides the other with enough space for their respective fields of interest. The husband encourages his wife to carry on her dancing lessons and she his public speaking. The point here is that the biggest destroyer of happy marriages is crowding the spousal space and not allowing each other enough freedom to grow.

The second destroyer of happy marriages is expecting your spouse to do what your parents were doing for each other. Here I will quote my example. My mother never started eating until my father was halfway through his meal. She never tasted a seasonal fruit until my father had tasted it first. I saw this from a very young age and formed a model of how a wife should behave. My wife came from a different background. I would find her licking her fingers, having finished her meal before I came home for lunch. She would gleefully tell me the mangoes were utterly delicious. This would upset me and I would sulk. It took me some years to deal with the issue.

In fact, it was a clash between two mental models and not a clash between two people. I finally realized that if I had the right to come into the marriage with a model of my own, then my wife had the same right. What gave me exclusive rights? With this insight, I dropped my expectations, not only in the matter of meals but also in other areas of our lives.

Another big destroyer of marriages is the sense of ownership – 'My husband/wife', 'How dare she/he do this?' We give enough liberty to our friends, but when it comes to our spouses, it is another story. This sense of ownership is a recipe for unhappiness. My experience as a marriage counsellor also tells me that couples spend a lot of time repairing/correcting the behaviour of others, through what psychologists call External Control Psychology. Let me tell you, external control or trying to correct the behaviour of others, does not work – it only seems to work. The partner goes into a shell and does what he wants to do, without sharing anything with the spouse.

Many times I am asked whether love marriages are more successful than arranged marriages. It is wise to break this myth. Love marriages are no more successful than arranged marriages. Talking of love marriage, we do not fall in love with anyone, we merely fall in love with the image of what another person should be like.

My experience as a counsellor also tells me that when things do not work in a marriage, the partners start blackmailing each other. The husband might say: 'If you don't listen to me I will not give you money'. The wife might respond: 'If you don't give me money I will not see to your comforts, physical or otherwise'. Some couples tell me, although they are unhappy in their marriage, they are staying in it for the sake of the children, believing that they are thereby doing the children a favour by sacrificing their own happiness. But research shows that children who are brought up in dysfunctional marriages are worse off than those who grow up with divorced parents. So my recommendation is to stay in marriage for the sake of yourself, and not make children or society the reason to continue in an unhappy marriage.

How is your Marriage Going?

Is there a test to know if one's marriage is happy or not? Yes, there is. When you can share your innermost thoughts and feelings with your spouse, without fear of rejection, blame, ridicule or complaint, you can say that you are living in a happy marriage.

What about divorce? Divorce is a legitimate way of ending a marriage if it is not working. It can be done in an adult, civilized and amicable manner. Once you have decided to separate, do you really want to throw mud at each other? How would that achieve your happiness and peace? Do not listen to friends who may give you a load of advice which cannot really help you. I recommend you take the help of a counsellor to guide you through this traumatic, painful period, and to deal with post-divorce adjustments.

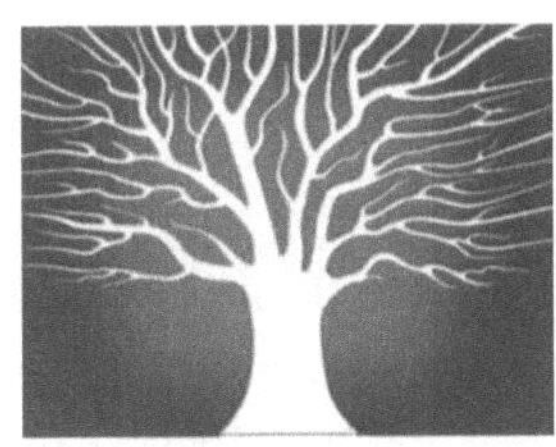

As a lay counsellor, I refuse to see any 'problem child' brought by their parents. Not until the parents have had a few sessions anyway. Sometimes the children are as young as six or seven, with a naughty glint in their eyes, and their parents want them to undergo therapy or counselling sessions!

Problem parents, yes; problem teachers, yes; problem society, yes; but problem children, no! To believe there are problem children is to believe children are born with a debased bent of mind or delinquency. If there is a problem child, there is a problem context in which he is being brought up. Change the quality of the environment and the child, over a period, will respond.

Experience shows that parents who bring their children for counselling, have a number of emotional issues themselves; this in turn affects the behaviour pattern of the child. In some cases, love is totally denied to the child who thinks: 'If I can't get love, I can get hate', and begins to behave in a delinquent manner. The common response to such behaviour is punishment. Unhappy homes produce unhappy children. What such children need is not therapy but the freedom to be themselves. Love, trust and freedom are the cure, not external discipline.

In schools, children are labelled hyperactive, slow, moody, not interested in mathematics, interested only in sports. And so on. Parents and teachers huddle in conference to find solutions to the problems they themselves have created through such mindless labelling of children. What such parents and teachers are doing is using the bar of

Problem Child? Not Really.

their own expectations of the child, who remains in the background. The fixed notions of adults become the main issues.

How often has one seen parents competing by pushing their children towards higher goals in areas the children themselves are not one bit interested in? The pity is that children are often compelled to fit into a system they are not in sync with. Then, of course, they become 'problem' children and need to be labelled. The pace at which each child develops becomes unimportant. That there are many children who bloom later than others, is forgotten. I know of a child who loves swimming but was sent to badminton coaching camps because the father was a former state badminton champion.

It is unfortunate that the bed wetting habit of a child is classified as a problem and a major topic of discussion between parents, their friends, and the grandparents. The parental concern is picked up by the child, who begins to feel guilty about something he is too young to have control over. The bed-wetting generates debate. Doctors are consulted. Some parents forget they themselves were also bed-wetters in childhood. Something which should be taken in their stride becomes a big 'problem'.

We often forget that a child is a dynamic entity with a young mind of his own. Adults believe a child's mind is a clean slate on which they can write their own scripts. The child is rarely allowed to live out his desires. Obedience is demanded without question. Discipline is ensured through punishment. Adult laws apply to them.

Why do we do this? I suspect it is because the most obvious scapegoat for the 'problem' is the child; he becomes the target and all attention is focussed on finding solutions for him rather than ourselves. It is convenient because other measures would require working on ourselves as parents, teachers and a nurturing society. Introspection is painful because it highlights chinks in us which we are not always ready to admit exist.

Problem Child? Not Really.

The question arises: Do not parents and teachers have a role in shaping the destiny of a child? Of course, they do. But that role is to provide security, appreciation and understanding of the child's own aspirations, which he tries to express but which, in the process of growing up, often gets suppressed.

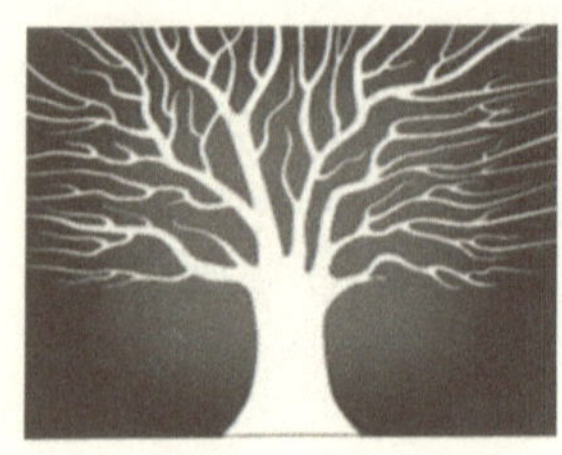

This is the cry of a counsellor – to parents, teachers, friends, relatives and neighbours. In fact, to anyone who cares to listen. Stop invalidating others under the guise of being well-wishers.

I had just returned from seeing Madhuri, a young girl of eighteen, who had tried to commit suicide a week earlier, by inflicting cuts on her wrists. She had been saved just in time because her mobile phone kept ringing, unanswered. Her brother, unable to bear the continuous ringing, barged into her room – to find her lying in a pool of blood. Madhuri was saved the indignity of the law taking its course by being treated by a doctor who was a relative.

Madhuri's doleful story began with these sobbed-out words: "I have no right to live, Uncle. I have no right to live. I am no good. I am no damn good. It is best that I disappear from this world." Most of her words were lost in her sobs but her pain was not. She thought she had no right to live because from early childhood, she had received one message: You are no good. Her mother continually said, "Look at your sister! How neat and clean she is. And look at you, you cry baby. Shame on you!"

The message from the schoolteacher was no less brutal an attack on Madhuri's self-esteem. She was hauled up for missing distinction by five marks. The fact that she had substantially improved upon her earlier performance was of little interest to the teacher. Her music instructor said: "I don't know why I am wasting time on you. You are not a patch on the other students."

Cry of a Counsellor

Young Madhuri lived in a joint family and her aunt would boast about the intellectual achievements of her children while making snide remarks about Madhuri. If she took the matter to her mother, she was told: "You can't complain about your aunt, you silly girl."

Madhuri went into a mild depression and was taken to a doctor: "He said that if I carried on like this, I would be a nervous wreck". The fact that she was one already, which is why she was there to consult with him, escaped the good practitioner. Madhuri told me that her self-esteem hit such a low that she would cross to the other side of the road when she saw people approaching. "What would they think of me?" she asked plaintively. She would slink out of the living room when guests arrived, because she felt she was not worth their company and attention. She would be severely reprimanded by her mother for being 'haughty' and leaving the room when guests came.

Deeply depressed, Madhuri decided that the pain of living was greater than the pain of dying – and attempted suicide. Her hopelessness now needed to be converted to hope through counselling. Madhuri is not alone in her struggle. Invalidation of the young means just one thing – they are destined to carry this heavy baggage throughout their lives; therefore, they hesitate to let anyone enter their world, worried their feelings will be brutalised again. They live in superficial relationships. One of the great leaders in education, Haim Ginnot, said: *'Primum non norce* (first do no harm)'. Do not wrong a teenager's perceptions. Do not argue with his experience. Do not disown his feelings. Ginnot would be disappointed to see his advice ignored so widely and repeatedly. Why am I making an issue against invalidation by citing just one case? This case is just a trigger. The malady lies deep in our society, where people criticise others instead of looking within.

Some of us counsellors had met for an informal chat and the conversation came round to the one big reason for the destruction of morale in the people who came to us for counselling. Since there was no single, ready answer, we began digging into the details of recent cases we had handled. In all cases, without exception, there was loss of self-esteem or lack of understanding by someone very close.

Invalidation is to reject, ignore, mock, tease or diminish someone's feelings. It can reach the stage when the person begins to feel not only invalidated but that there is something fundamentally wrong with him. Psychological invalidation is the most lethal form of emotional abuse. The language of invalidation is so commonplace it can be uttered without understanding the damage involved: 'You are over reacting'; 'Stop being a jerk'; 'You need to have your head examined'; 'What is the problem with you?'; 'Look at your brother, he is so intelligent'. Do I need to go on with the language of rejection when we already have mastery over it? Telling someone he should not feel the way he does, is akin to telling water it should not be wet, or telling the grass it should not be green, or a rock that it should not be hard. To that person, his feelings are real and that is the only thing that matters to him. And that is the only thing we need to acknowledge.

I look around and see so much emotional terrorism of youngsters going on, in the name of helping them to cope with this terrible world – parental and teacher terrorism. And the resulting invalidation makes those children suffer throughout their lives.

So, I go back to where we began. This is the cry of a lay counsellor to whoever cares to listen – stop invalidating others.

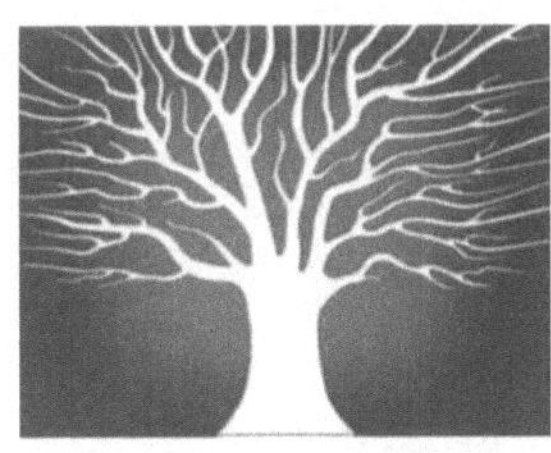

As a counsellor, it came as a surprise to discover that low self-esteem was one of the most common emotional issues I would be dealing with. Roughly, one in four who come to me for counselling suffer from unhappiness caused by low self-esteem (depression being another common emotional trauma). I don't think that corporate chiefs have ever applied themselves to the economic loss a company suffers because a fair percentage of their people are producing far less than their capability, because they think they are not people of worth and dignity. Twenty-five percent lowered productivity of a machine would set alarm bells ringing in a factory; but the same loss in human terms goes unnoticed. A broken human spirit is rarely seen and fixed but a broken machine certainly is.

What are the signs of low self-esteem? Human issues cannot be put into a box and labelled neatly. People with low self-esteem can generally be said to have a low self-worth and sense of dignity. They torment themselves and miss out on the joy in their lives. They get into self-bashing moods; while they might show understanding of others' shortcomings, they apply harsh standards to themselves. In general, they go through life in bitterness, frustration and disillusionment.

The root cause of low self-esteem is negative thoughts that produce bad feelings. The way these negative thoughts are handled compounds the problem. The people who come for counselling keep trying to push out their negative thoughts and conquer them. However, the more they persist with this exercise, the more the negative thoughts resist, and a vicious circle develops. Unfortunately, only a few such people reach out for therapeutic counselling. It is recommended that those who feel hopeless and overwhelmed and cannot relate to others in a positive way, would fare better if they sought counselling from a trained person.

It is my experience that sometimes better results have been achieved through the spiritual approach than the psychological approach, although the latter is also effective with some. Acceptance of oneself as one is and not considering low self-esteem as something shameful or unusual, itself releases a lot of negative energy. The reason it works is that the mind is not divided into different segments – one producing negative thoughts and the other fighting those thoughts. 'This is how it is with me at this time', is a statement which brings peace and healing; one is then able to see one's position more clearly. The realization that one is a human being with human fallings, and that does not mean that one is a defective person, lifts a heavy burden from the mind. Good counsellors are alert to the possibility of this approach being misunderstood though, when people try to embrace their shortcomings in a bid to avoid facing and tackling them.

On a psychological or mental level, if one can gain freedom from the curse of 'should', many issues can be resolved: 'I am such a fool; I shouldn't have made such a silly mistake'; 'I should be as good as my colleague'; 'I should have more self-confidence at my age and with my experience'. Such 'should' thoughts make mincemeat of one's self-esteem. Try replacing 'should' with 'would/could', to describe the same situation: 'It would have been far better if I had prepared myself better' or 'I could try to do it differently the next time'.

The other thing that comes in the way of dealing with low self-esteem, is that such people are unduly harsh on themselves. In the process, they tend to generalise their faults. 'I am a total failure', they will tell themselves, rather than looking at specific strengths and weaknesses. They are generous with others in accommodating weaknesses but not with themselves. Then they display double standards, reserving harsher standards for themselves. Once they achieve an understanding

Dealing with Low Self-Esteem

of the root cause of their negative thoughts which evoke negative feelings, the process of recovery begins.

It is helpful to realize the mood we create is an internal process. People with low self-esteem sometimes get into a victim mode and begin to believe the source of their misery lies out there with that person or that happening. They are quite happy complaining about how bad things are as long as they do not have to do anything to solve their problems. There is hope for such people if they can be guided to look at themselves as the source and realise that the only control we have is over how we respond to situations around us. The most important factor to recovery is to move away from the victim mode and take charge. This is a painful process but the necessary cost a person must be willing to pay to regain his sense of worth and dignity. Dr David D Burns says that bad feelings are often caused by distorted thoughts. When you put the lie to these distorted thoughts, you can *change* the way you feel.

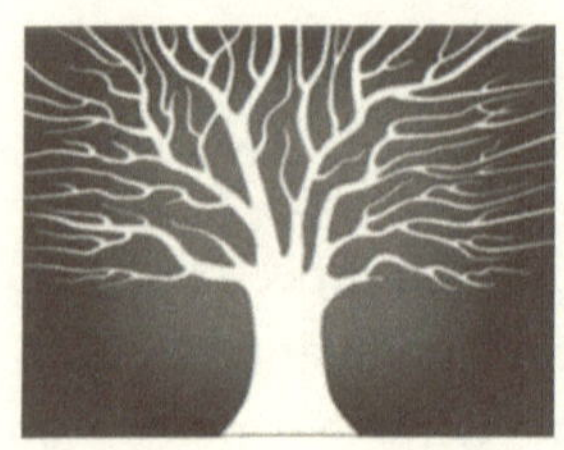

Marital music can be as uplifting as a symphony, a pleasure to be enjoyed. It can also comprise the most jarring notes. What causes the difference? The most common reason is expectations, with a capital E. The worst of marital expectations is that spouses assume the other partner knows what the expectations are, even when unexpressed. There are many reasons for marital disharmony but number one on the list would perhaps be an unstated list of expectations.

In marital counselling, we invite couples to look at this aspect of living and see if they can clearly put on the table what their expectations of the other are. The next step is to negotiate those expectations and establish those that fall into the doable category and those that are non-negotiable. Often the response is: 'I did not know you wanted this. Why did you not tell me before?' Seeking mutual agreement is the most difficult part of alignment in marriage since the positions have already hardened over time.

There is another myth about marriage, which is that the longer a marriage has survived, the happier it is. In reality, it is often seen that major differences in married life surface as the couple grows older. The reason is that at some point in their growth as individuals, the pace of growth or the routes to growth, become different. One of the partners may be attracted toward spirituality while the other may enjoy kitty parties. One spouse may think; 'What is left to be done now that I am nearly sixty?' while the other thinks the fun and games have just started now that the children are settled.

Marital Music

If there are signs of marital discord, it is best to seek the help of a trained counsellor. Discussing it with friends is not recommended because experience shows that friends become like the seconds to two heavyweight boxers. You can almost hear, 'Seconds out of the ring, first round time'. Besides, friends carry their own marital ideas, which are often infectious. This may seem like stating the obvious, but it needs to be underscored as an important point. There is yet another danger – even if our own marriage is in a mess, we still believe we can fix others' marriages. There are as many opinions on repairing marriages as the number of friends you seek help from, leaving you even more confused. Counsellors too, often have these notions and get into advisory mode.

The intensity of problems in marriage increases logarithmically as there are two individuals involved. What kind of issues does one see in cases of marital discord? In fact, every issue tied to and caused by human frailty. Money, sex, extra-marital affairs, physical and verbal abuse are the most common. Even when few expectations remain, remember to bring these out into the open and negotiate them.

The best marriage advice comes from Khalil Gibran in *The Prophet*:

But let there be spaces in your togetherness
And let the winds of heaven dance between you
Love one another, but make not a bond of love
Let it rather be a moving sea between the shores of your souls
Fill each other's cup but drink not from one cup
Give one another of your bread but not from the same loaf
Sing and dance together and be joyous, but let each one of be alone
Even as the strings of lute are alone though they quiver with the same music
Give your hearts, but not into each other's keeping
For only the hand of life can contain your hearts
And stand together and not near together

For the pillars of temples stand apart.
And the oak tree and Cyprus grow not in each other's shadow.

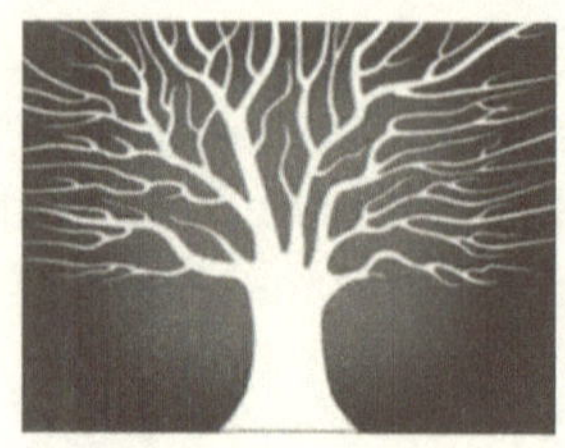

The three Cs – criticism, condemnation and comparison – in childhood, can cause havoc in adulthood. An earlier chapter had the case of a young 18-year-old who was utterly condemned, ruthlessly compared and severely criticized, and chose to attempt suicide. I do not for a moment suggest the parents did so by design. Rather, by default. If one were to look back, it would be no surprise to find they themselves were the victims of victims. Their parents compared, condemned and criticised them in childhood and they perpetuated this behaviour in the next generation. It might be worthwhile to examine what other wounds we parents/adults can cause our children. These are sometimes called primal wounds.

The first primal wound is *engulfment*. Here, the parents are so intrusive, overbearing and overpowering that there is little space given to the child to grow on his own. They crowd the child in two ways. The first is to overwhelm the child by meeting all his needs, whether those needs are appropriate for his age or not. All this is done in the name of love. The other way is to engulf through physical abuse and domineering behaviour, in the name of discipline. Children who are engulfed are non self-starters when they grow up. Either they grow up thinking the world owes them everything or they need to be kicked around to move them to achieve something, because they were not allowed any space in their childhood.

The second primal wound is *abandonment*. Some children hate to be in boarding schools. But parents, in their wisdom, think boarding school will make a man out of the child and, much against his wishes, send the child away. He feels abandoned: 'My parents do not need me'. He

Primal Wounds

grows up to be untrusting: 'I could not trust my parents to take care of me. Why should I trust this person or society?'

The third primal wound we inflict on children is *hurt*. When parents/ adults cannot deal with their own emotional problems, they project those problems onto their children by physically, emotionally and even sexually abusing them. Such children, when they grow up, cannot have deep and lasting relationships because they fear that they may get hurt. They generally have poor marriages because they are apprehensive they may get hurt in the relationship.

And the last primal wound is *non-involvement*, where parents are physically present but do not make any emotional connection with the child. They are there and yet not there because they are self-absorbed. The child feels emotionally abandoned.

Why these details? Because I believe we love our children. We want to do the very best for them but unfortunately, out of love but also out of ignorance, we end up achieving exactly the opposite result to that intended. We may have been the victims of our parents, who were victims of their parents – but is there any need to maintain that negative course?

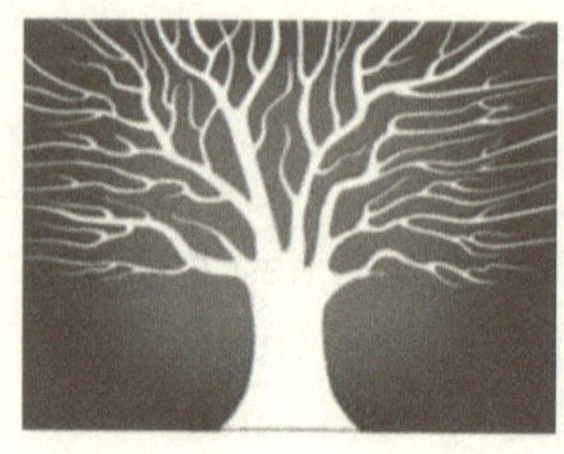

We live in an age of anxiety; its sceptre hangs over us constantly, the basis of many mental health issues. Mental health professionals are deeply concerned about the future, in which depression and anxiety are poised to be major issues. We are talking here of 8-10% of our population suffering from disabling and neurotic anxiety. Translate this into actual figures and you get an idea of the severity of the issue.

Normal anxiety

Like stress, you can have normal and abnormal levels of anxiety. If someone is not well at home, of course you will be anxious. If you are a student, it is quite normal to be anxious before exams. If a marriage is under strain, there will be attendant anxiety for the couple. It would be abnormal if you did not feel anxious before a major surgery. I personally feel anxious when I leave home for a holiday, only to enjoy myself once I have reached the destination.

Abnormal anxiety

Here we are talking about abnormal anxiety of the type when life loses its colour, resulting in insomnia, palpitations, and accelerated pulse. You feel queasy. There is a sense of panic and you break into an embarrassing sweat. I have experienced this when asked to address a group. Abnormal anxiety also visits us as nightmares or when you feel anxious but do not even know the reason why. Underlying anxiety is fear of something external or internal. Or shall we say fear is the context for this type of anxiety.

You would know mothers who stand at the gate, waiting for the school bus to arrive; if it is more than ten minutes late, panic buttons get pressed. These excessive anxieties turn a normal person into a neurotic one. It gets worse if you cannot find an outlet to express the anxiety. Tranquilisers provide temporary relief but soon the panic attacks revisit us with greater ferocity than before.

Phobic disorders

There are some among us who have irrational fears of dogs, lizards, heights, lifts, closed-doors or air travel. Some have phobias about social settings, being alone, walking alone on a street, and other irrational fears that just do not go away. The worst is that we cannot even describe these fears accurately and when we can, we get buck-up and shake-out-of-it calls from well-meaning family and friends. Well intentioned they are, but they do not realize the inner voice of an anxious person speaks a different message. The first thing to remember is: *Never challenge the reality of the anxious.*

Who is more susceptible?

Experience shows that anxiety most often attacks the introverted, who cannot express themselves fully and prefer to resolve all their issues by themselves. It also visits those who have a negative bent of mind and find a dark side to everything they see. Additionally, it affects people who lack a strong coping mechanism. For example, it is now established by the medical community that regular exercise is a very effective antidote for anxiety. Those with an exaggerated notion of their capabilities or those who believe they have not received due recognition of their abilities, are more prone to anxiety.

Anxiety is treatable

The good news is that anxiety is treatable. As a counsellor, I have often seen bouts of anxiety dissipate because the anxious person is able to share and express their fears to a counsellor who is willing to listen, understand and empathise – not sermonise. Some abnormal cases do need to be treated by a psychologist or psychiatrist, supported by a counsellor to whom they can vent their thoughts and feelings during

The Scepter of Anxiety

the period the medical professionals are managing the illness with the help of medication.

This may sound simplistic but what works for me is to observe my anxiety and not struggle to evict it. I find that anxiety, like an uninvited guest, goes away. But if I try to shoo it away, it becomes more determined and almost dares me to blink first. In that mode, I usually do.

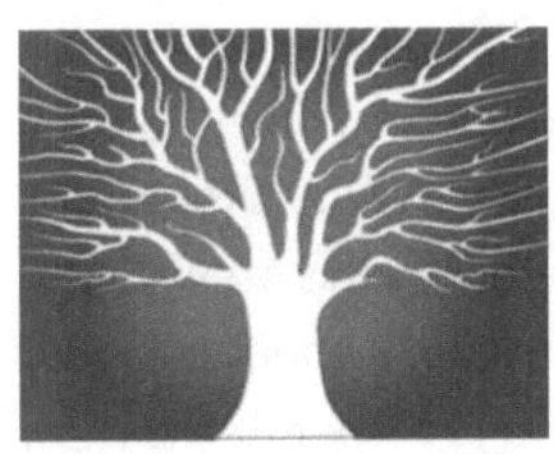

In the course of his research about the reasons for divorce, a practising divorce lawyer set up a meeting with me to get a counsellor's prospective. During our freewheeling conversation, I emphasised my belief that it is usually a clash between the quality worlds of the partners that rocks the marriage boat. What is this quality world? The following examples will explain the concept.

Lata was brought up in a family where boys and girls were treated equally and there was freedom of expression. If, at a young age, Lata needed money, she would explain the need to her mother who would hand over the keys of the cupboard to her and trust Lata to take the agreed amount. Exactly the opposite was the case with her husband, Sunil. He was brought up with strict controls, where he had not only to fight for every rupee, but when the allowance was grudgingly granted, his father would pull out his wallet and count the money twice before handing it over to his son.

Lata and Sunil grew up in different quality worlds in how to deal with monetary demands from their children. Lata would do what she had seen her mother do and Sunil would follow the script embedded on his hard disc. This became a source of constant bickering: 'You careless woman,' "You stingy man, escalated to: 'You irresponsible woman! I work my bottom off to earn, and here you go spending money like water'. Soon four letter words were flying between them in their destructive dialogues.

Let us look at another example of the clash of quality worlds. The husband came from a family where his father was the sole decision-maker – from which curtains would adorn the hall to what would be the budget for each category of expense. All hell broke loose if the rules of the game were violated. Even minor infringements were not tolerated. In short, it was my-way-or-the-highway approach. On the other hand, the wife came from a family where her father's salary cheque would be deposited into a joint account, which was mostly operated by her mother. Her father was busy with his work and if details were offered, he would ask his wife to leave him alone and manage the way she wanted to. Their varying childhood scripts were so heavily imprinted upon their minds that the couple found the behaviour of each other absolutely unacceptable.

The lawyer looked at me in disbelief and asked: "Do you mean to say that husbands and wives have to be clones of each other for a happy marriage? Are you saying we are carbon copies of our parents?" He obviously found such propositions farfetched. A little known fact of psychology is that what we become as adults is largely influenced by childhood scripts. For example, if a child grows up in an environment of criticism, comparison and condemnation, he is most likely to grow up to be a person of low self-esteem and have difficulty in experiencing the fullness of a married relationship or other relationships. The child who receives unconditional love grows up to be comfortable and secure in a loving relationship. The child who grows up with parents who rush to meet his every whim, grows up believing the world owes him the same kind of response. In this respect, we are the victims of victims. Our parents saw their parents behave in a certain way, and believing that was the right way, perpetuated identical behaviour patterns with their children. These childhood primal scars or invalidations have a lot to do with what we turn out to be – hostile and untrusting or loving and generous.

Also, do not forget the genes effect. While the debate about nature (genes) or nurture (upbringing), carries on, let us remember that parents provide both nature and nurture. That is not to say individuals cannot break the vicious circle of generations but it takes effort, which requires inquiry, which needs asking: 'Who am I being in this relationship? Is there a better way?' This kind of thinking requires work and therefore the vast majority of us continue to live our childhood scripts unless we are kicked where it hurts. One such husband who came in for counselling, began to see his wife's point of view when she said there was no way she would live in an abusive marriage. He woke up to the reality of their marriage and modified his behaviour.

On the subject of husbands and wives being clones of each other, I will say that cloning does not mean similar behaviour. But to some extent, it does mean a similar set of values. For instance, if I have the right to grow in the field of my interest, so has my wife the right to pursue what she enjoys. If my values are important to me, her values are equally important to her.

The space to grow at an individual pace in a chosen sphere, is an important aspect of happy marriages. The divergence of the quality worlds of the spouses also reflects on the health of their marriage. At the end of the day, it is the overlap or divergence of the quality worlds of the spouses that determines success or failure in marriage.

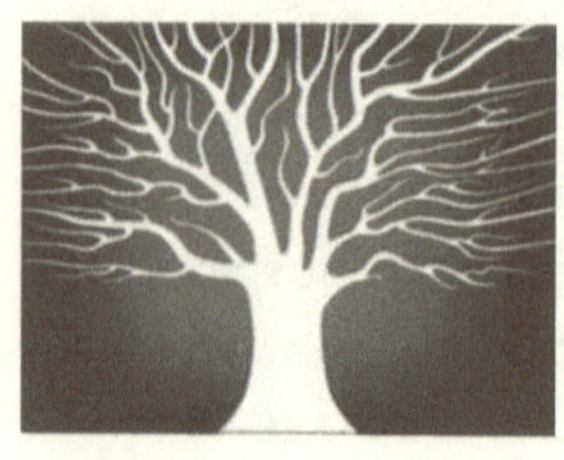

Falling in love and getting married is easy. Staying in love and staying happily married is a darn sight more difficult. As a counsellor, I have seen many couples lamenting the current state of their marriage. Many of them were madly in love when they took the decision to get married. This certainly needs some explanation.

When you are blindly in love, you are just that – blind. You are in a state of emotionality, unable to think clearly. The caste, creed, height, colour, waistline, bustline and religion of the object of your affections do not matter. Your personal ego boundaries collapse before the other person's. You merge with each other. You are, to use a local expression common in south India, one-by-two coffee. The conversation goes like this: 'Where shall we go out to eat?' 'Anywhere you like.' You reach the restaurant and the first question is: 'Darling, what would you like to eat?' The answer usually is" 'Whatever you order'. This is honeymoon talk. But this is nothing but hormones playing tricks. *Beware*!

Soon the honeymoon is over. You start regaining your ego boundaries. You become you and she becomes she. Now the same person begins to crowd your personal space. Both of you regain your personal ego states, your individuality, and your boundaries. Social norms begin to raise their ugly head.

However much we deny the fact, my experience in counselling couples convinces me that we have been and continue to be, a male dominated society. I have known husbands to say jocularly, but mean seriously, that a woman's place is in the kitchen and bedroom (in that order). This societal view of marriage is the source of much marital discord.

When Deep in Love, Do Not Marry

I raise a question here which you do not need to answer but should certainly reflect upon: When things are not working well in a marriage, who is generally given the freewheeling advice – husband or wife? I am willing to go along with the assertion that things change; but how fast are they changing? I believe that for any change to last, the process needs to evolutionary, not revolutionary. These are real life marriage issues. You can wish them away only at your personal peril. Being in love is hard work. Being in love requires discipline that allows the other space to grow. And our childhood image of marriage constantly tests that discipline.

A personal example will help. My father gave all he earned to my mother. He left her to manage the home finances. I did exactly the same. My wife manages the accounts. There is no divergence here from my model and therefore no sulking. Here, my quality world matches that of my wife. It is when there is a divergence and dispersion in the quality worlds of the spouses that the maximum damage is caused in a marriage. And it carries on until you ask yourself this question: 'Where in the world did I get the right to expect my wife should behave in a particular way?'

We may not be ready to admit it but I do not think many of us would disagree that it is in marriage that the concept of ownership is the strongest. The same person you were showing off when she was your fiancée, as the best waltz dancer in the city, becomes the source of jealousy when she dances with your best friend post-marriage. Then the blackmail starts: 'If you carry on like this, I will cut off your finances', 'If it were not for you, I would not have this drinking problem'. Then the couple goes into a passive state. Live and let live becomes the rule of the game. Mending the marriage or breaking it, both require will, which is usually not forthcoming. Of course, you find sacrificial reasons like for-the-sake-of-the-children…

Marriage is as risky a business as the stock market. The *mentex* of marriage fluctuates as frequently as the sensex, except that the exit

When Deep in Love, Do Not Marry

options or handing over the portfolio to a fund manager, is not an option in marriage. The stakes are high, so enter the institution of marriage with your eyes wide open. Project your future with that person; see the context of their childhood (very important); and how the family treats one another. Are their value systems in sync with yours? Do I mean that the person be your clone? Not at all. But certainly a person who will allow you the space to grow mentally, emotionally and spiritually. I have left out physically. That is the easy part because hormones and genes take care of it. Romance and love are two different matters. For romance, log onto www.Bollywoodsongs.com and www. Bollywoodmovies.com – for the biggest delusions of what marriage is.

Marriage is a serious business. Khalil Gibran, in his must-read book *The Prophet*, reminds us that love is not velvety smooth; the other side is abrasive rock.

When love beckons to you, follow him,
Though his ways are hard and steep.
And when his wings enfold you yield to him,
Though the sword hidden among his pinions may wound you.
And when he speaks to you believe in him.
Though his voice may shatter your dreams
as the north wind lays waste the garden...

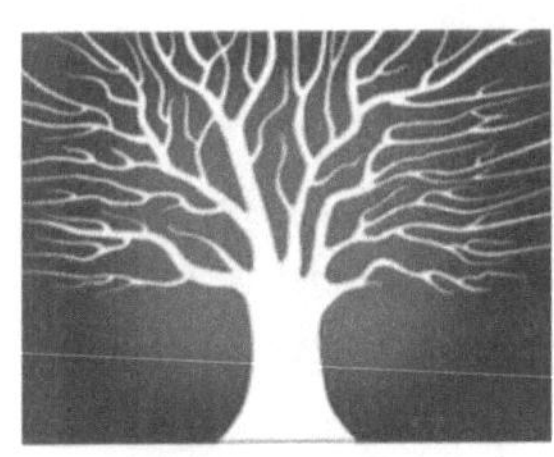

Suppose you could ask those people who are not hungry, sick, or poor, and seem to have a lot to live for, to give you an honest answer to the question, 'How are you?', what would they say? Millions would tell you, 'I am miserable and unfulfilled'. Almost all would blame someone else for their misery – lovers, wives, husbands, children, parents, teachers, students or people they work with. There are few people who have not said, 'You are driving me crazy! Your behaviour really upsets me. Don't you have any consideration for how I feel?' or 'You make me so mad, I can't even think straight'.

Little do we realize, that for all practical purposes it is we who choose everything, including the misery we feel. Other people cannot make us feel miserable or happy. All we can get from them or give them is information. By itself, information cannot make us do or feel anything. It is just raw information. It goes into the brain where we process it and then decide what we will do with it. That is the moment when we can exercise the Power of Choice. Each choice we make creates an experience for us and for others. That choice lies with us, it is in our control and no one can take that control from us unless we surrender it.

Let me give you a personal example of how I chose to be miserable for a whole day. It is a habit with me to fill myself up with salads, vegetables and lentils. Months go by when I have not touched rice, *chapati* or bread. It is what I have chosen to do, but it is not a hard and fast rule. Last week for instance, I made an exception and said to my wife: "You know, I loved those Kerala *parathas* Meera served at her house. Do you know from where she gets them? Could you get some when you go for your music class?" My wife replied: "She did mention something but I have forgotten the name of the shop." I then said: "Why don't you call her and find out where she got them from?" This was my wife's reply: "You want Kerala *parathas*, you ring up Meera and find out where she got them from." I asked: "Why can't you do it for me?" To which she replied impatiently: "Okay *baba*, okay."

Sounds familiar? That did it for me and I said to myself, 'Look at her. She knows that I don't touch these things for months together. And today, when I thought I would enjoy some *parathas*, this is the answer I get. The least she can do is find out and get them for me'.

I went into a miserable sulk of Himalayan proportions. I stomped out of the room, did not talk to her for the whole day, and kept saying to myself that it was awful on her part to respond like that. The long and short of it was that I spent a whole day feeling miserable because I chose misery. I thought I would show her but it was exactly the opposite. She said, did and behaved in her usual way. I was powerless. But what about myself? My response had been in my control and what a miserable choice I had made. There was no one to clean up the mess but me.

I will go a step further and say that the way we see ourselves is also a choice. Do we perceive ourselves as beautiful or ugly? Do we view ourselves as smart or stupid, handsome or plain, inferior or superior? It is our choice. In fact, we can simply say our choices equal our creations. If we do not like the creation or the consequences of it, we have to look at the choices that created the consequence.

If we do not realize that our experiences are the consequences of our choices, we will continue to believe that others are what we perceive them to be – just or unjust, good or bad. We will continue to be rudderless boats, tossed helplessly by the crashing waves, and feel victimised by others. But once the connection between our choices and our experiences is established in the mind, we can avoid creating the same experience again.

Choose Happiness

We also come across people who, in a similar situation, act very differently. The difference lies in the choices they have made. If you have experienced misery with your spouse, bosses, colleagues or friends, it is most likely that one of the following four variations of attempting to control someone, is taking place:

- *You* wanted someone to do something; that person refused. You were trying to dominate someone and they said: 'Get off my back'.
- Someone was trying to make *you* do something you did not want to do. In other words, someone was trying to dominate you and you were saying; 'Get off my back'.
- Both *someone* and *you* wanted to make each other do something neither wanted to do.
- *You* were trying to force yourself to do something painful or impossible to do.

As long as we continue to believe we can control others or others can control us, misery will result. This is worse in close relationships with spouses, children or old friends. Then another angle comes in – ownership. 'How can my wife refuse to do what I ask?' 'My children had better listen to me.' Observe that you do not have great expectations from a stranger because there is no ownership in the mind. So let us understand that feelings of misery or happiness are within us. Others sing their own songs and create their drama. But we feel miserable because we make that choice. Therefore we must own responsibility for making it.

There is another thing we do and that is to play rackets (I have dwelt at length on the concept of 'rackets' earlier in the book). A 'racket' is being something or doing something and continuously complaining – such as being in a marriage, working with a boss, doing something your friends want but you do not want – and continuing to complain. Year after year. This is a common behaviour we use to shift the blame onto someone else for our misery. People keep complaining about

Choose Happiness

someone for 20 years and still carry on in that relationship. After a while, we begin to enjoy the victim's role, along with the sympathy and attention we get. We enjoy hearing, 'Poor thing'. We have to stop playing rackets. Either we say we will not submit to the indignity being heaped upon us, or we stop complaining.

Stephen Covey puts it neatly when he says that the word 'responsibility' is really two words, 'respond' and 'ability'. It is all about our ability to respond. What others say or do are just stimuli. We have no control over that. We can only control the response to the stimulus. That is our choice. We can retaliate, disengage, sleep over it, deal with compassion or negotiate. But we cannot spend our lives repairing the issue. That is a zero-sum, tiring, non-winnable game. That is a game played by the irresponsible.

People with a scientific bent of mind believe in cause and effect theory. If they do not like the effect, they start looking at the cause. It is the same in our lives. If you do not like the effect, consequence or experience, look at the choice that caused it. If we maintain the same choice, we can be sure we will continue to undergo the same experience. When we choose differently, we create differently.

Coming back to the Kerala *parathas* incident, which generated so much anger in me – looking back, it was the result of the choice I made. I could certainly have chosen differently and rung up our friend and found out about the source of the *parathas*. I could have sent my driver and got them for both of us to enjoy. What I did instead was place myself in a self-constructed behaviour-prison. I became the prisoner. And I was the only one who could set myself free. The ball was in my court.

Waking up to personal choices in life is a powerful way to live.

Choose Happiness

POSTSCRIPT

You get in touch with the finest example of making a choice when you read Victor Frankle's book, *Life's Search for Meaning*. Victor Frankle was an Austrian Jew and a psychiatrist, who was imprisoned by Hitler's army. Along with other prisoners, he was made to do the most horrific, life-threatening tasks in extreme weather conditions, on meagre food, facing constant degradation. Some of the prisoners would tell on their co-prisoners in order to get softer jobs or an extra slice of bread or a cigarette. But Victor would say to himself: 'You can take away my liberty and confine me in shackles but you cannot take away my freedom to think and act'. Choice Theory comes out so beautifully at the end of his book when he says: 'There were those amongst us who helped the Germans to build gas chambers and there were also those amongst us who walked into them with their heads held high'.

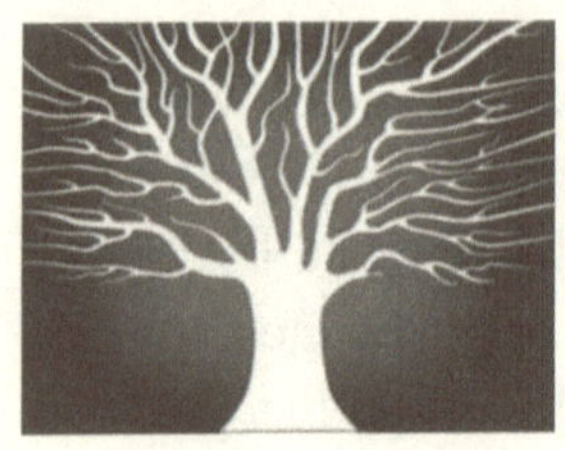

I never used to know what to say to someone who had lost a dear one. It was a problem I faced for years. I desperately wanted to offer condolences but would hold back, not knowing what the appropriate thing to say was. It got so bad I would avoid meeting those who were grieving, frozen by the fear of saying something inadequate. That was till I got married and learnt from my wife how to communicate with a grieving family. She taught me that time passes slowly when grief is fresh. Condolences are most comforting when offered as soon as one hears the sad news. It is not eloquence that is needed. An empathic touch to reinforce human contact is enough to express compassion and share grief.

Listening to those in mourning can provide more solace than talking. There is no need to ask questions. The words will come as part of the venting of their grief, if we but patiently listen. All we need to do is convey our willingness to hear. Allow the silences to be; they too are needed for the mind to find equilibrium. Don't rush to fill the pauses with inanities that have no meaning in that moment. When you say, "Time is the greatest healer', remember that, for the other person, time has stopped, it is cruel. So just be with them in empathy.

You cannot minimize someone's loss by saying 'You have other children' or 'It was destiny'. All that is meaningless noise to the grieving family. So just listen. There are a few other expressions that are irrelevant to a grieving family, the most commonly being: 'Her time had come' or 'It is best to remember the good times you had together' or 'God in His wisdom knows best'. Those grieving are not interested in such intellectual statements. They want to share their

Sharing Grief

feelings of pain, dejection, helplessness, and even anger. We can help more through actions than words. Bringing food, looking after a baby, making calls to those who need to know about the tragedy, are some things we can do.

In times of loss, the immediate family, friends and neighbours rush to condole but there remains is a vacuum after everyone has left. This is the time to revisit and be in touch on the phone. Sometimes we tend to overcrowd the grieving person with too frequent visits. They know you care. Be sensitive to the fact that sooner or later, they must return to their normal routine. Life goes on…

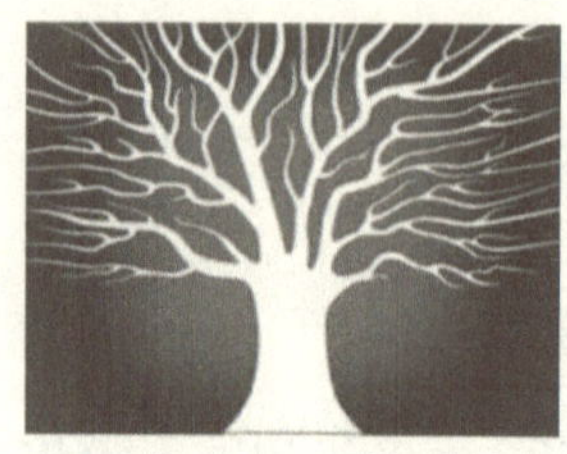

There are many societal issues that lie buried under the surface and need to be brought out into the open of general awareness. Child Sexual Abuse (CSA) is one of them. Indian society, by and large, is in a state of denial that this social problem exists. Therefore, even the shocking fact that abuse occurs with every other girl-child, and one in six boys, is either ignored or glossed over. Here, we look at some of the issues regarding abused children as well as adults who were abused as children.

If the abuse is currently going on, we have to do everything in our power to stop it – which usually means removing the child from the abusive situation. Often, the trauma stops during childhood but resurfaces later as the cause of adult problems. In some cases the child grows out of the abusive experience and learns to live a normal life. Despite the bad experiences such children are still able to trust people. They have suffered but have not been permanently damaged. But in about 20% of cases, the trauma continues into adulthood.

The aggressors are generally people the children trust and include the natural parents, uncles, cousins, neighbours or even teachers and religious heads. The biggest casualty of such abuse is trust, as the people most trusted are themselves the abusers. Children usually do not know how to handle the situation and often keep the experience of abuse to themselves. Distrustful, they remain in a prison of silence.

Apart from the total loss of trust, CSA manifests itself in many other ways like difficulty in entering into intimate relationships, anxiety, depression, shame, guilt and anger. It is shame and guilt, accompanied by a sense of entrapment, that keeps them in a shell of misery from which they find it difficult to break out; and the problem perpetuates.

Child Sexual Abuse & The Aftermath

The survivors of CSA may accidentally reveal the story or intentionally bring it to light because they want to deal with the painful and traumatic experience. The worst thing to do in such cases is to blame the person by saying things like: 'It must have been your fault', 'You are no good', 'Why did you allow such a thing to happen?' 'Why did you not tell me this before?' Such responses makes an already guilt-ridden person feel even more ashamed.

And the other thing to remember is that most of us are not equipped to handle CSA cases by ourselves. The only course of action is to seek counselling from an experienced person. During the counselling process, survivors are made to see that they are not suffering so much from the abuse itself as from the fact that they have lost trust in people. Mistrust makes sense to them in their experience. If they have been hurt by people who were role models, close relations, or neighbours, how can they possibly trust total strangers? What they have to understand is that most people are not abusers and most (not all), people can be trusted. They have to learn to distinguish those who can be trusted from those who cannot and stay clear of the second category. They have to be extra cautious to avoid being hurt again and lose the fragile trust they have begun to gain.

There are two schools of thoughts towards the counselling approach itself. One recommends revisiting the scene of the 'crime' by talking about the abuse history. This theory believes in going back in memory to create an acceptance of the history. Personally, I do not see much merit in this approach. Everything that we wish to change is in the present and therefore, revisiting a bad experience does not make the person stronger. William Glasser, in his book *Choice Theory*, puts it clearly, using a perfect analogy: If you have been starving for a long time, you need food, not an explanation why you were not fed in the past. Psychological wounds can be healed through understanding and love. Trusting relationships can be built again. Admittedly, an abused person, because of an unhappy past, may be less capable (not incapable), of dealing with the present. But this is true of all cases that enter the counselling process, regardless of the issues being dealt with. The past does not interfere with the present unless we make the choice to live in the past. That is what needs to be emphasized to the survivors of abuse.

What should family or caregivers do when they stumble upon, accidentally or intentionally, a case of child abuse? First and foremost, ensure the child is never again put into a situation where such abuse is possible. Look out for any behaviour patterns which may indicate any of the psychological effects mentioned in this chapter. If such abuse only comes to your notice when the person has reached adulthood, guide them to a reputed counselling centre. Also, in CSA cases, the family must make a point of enquiring into the experience of the counsellor in dealing with such cases. Not all counsellors are trained to handle CSA cases. Asking about the credentials of the counsellor is your right and you should exercise it.

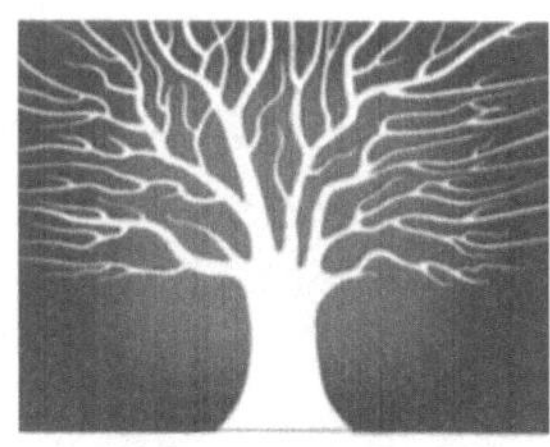

At this point, some readers may begin to have questions about their own mental health. 'How do I know I am mentally healthy?' is a valid doubt. Check yourself against the points below and you will get an indication about your mental health:

- What do you think of yourself? Is your self-image largely positive?
- Do you think you have the self-confidence to express your views and your feelings?
- Do you take responsibility for your actions and not see yourself as a victim of circumstances?

If you have inner strength and a sense of humour, you can celebrate and say to yourself, 'Of course, I am mentally healthy'. My gut feeling is that you are in a minority. Read on and then decide.

One should not take it for granted that once mentally healthy, always mentally healthy. In much the same way that we cannot take physical health for granted, we cannot take mental health as given. For physical health, you go for a walk; for mental health, you read books that keep you excited and make you want to turn to the next page. For physical health, you eat good, nourishing food; for mental health, you keep good, nurturing company. For physical health, you rest and relax; for mental health, you meditate and keep periods of silence. Eventually, each one finds a way to stay on the course of mental health. For physical health, you build stamina by being regular in your routine. It is the same with mental health, in order to build a stronger coping mechanism.

Mental Health Indicators

Here is another checklist given by Carkhuff that might help you to know where you stand on mental health: If you are frequently sad, or feel resentment, experience anxiety bouts, guilt, anger or rejection, things are probably not working for you in the area of mental health.

We function at different levels and this gives us a fix on where we stand on the issues of life.

- The lowest level is being a *detractor*. These are the people who look for the little black dot on an otherwise white and shining canvas. When you give them a bowl of well-prepared soup, they will say it should have been thicker, have more salt, or taste better than it does.
- The next level is that of the *observer*. He merely observes what is going on, and has no suggestions or contributions to make. These people get up in the morning with no agenda and live life listlessly and without excitement.
- The next level is that of the *participant*. Such people play the game according to the role assigned to them and do their best to play the ball when it is in their field.
- The next level is the *contributor*. Such people contribute with suggestions, effort, wealth and means, and volunteer to take more responsibility.
- The highest level is that of the *leader*. Such people lead from the front as captain of a team; they lead groups; give credit to the team when things go right; and take responsibility when things go wrong.

What do clients expect? This is what my experience tells me about client expectations:

- 'I am going to a counsellor and he will solve my problems and give me an easy QED solution'. They do not realize that the change has to happen from within and that change can only be assisted in some way by a counsellor.
- 'At least the counsellor will be able to put some sense into these nuts.' They do not realize that councellors cannot change

Mental Health Indicators

anyone's behaviour; they only have control over how they respond to what others do or say.

- 'I will get the counsellor's backing that I am on the right track and the reassurance that nothing will go wrong.'

Experienced counsellors do not demolish the expectations of clients, but through therapy sessions, the clients themselves begin to get in touch with reality and start looking at counsellors as the empathetic facilitators they are

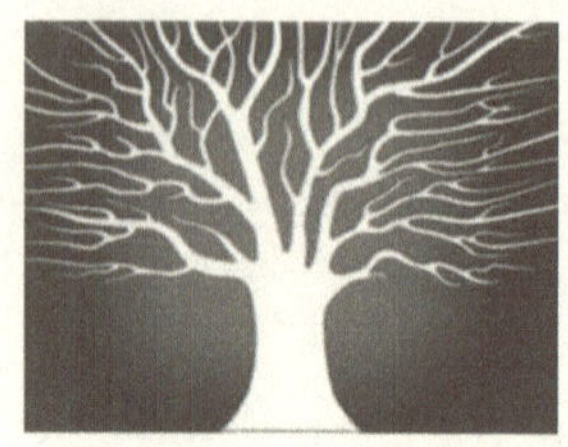

All professions (except politics), have an established code of conduct. So do counsellors. These are the norms by which we judge our behaviour. These norms have been derived from current social and moral values in society.

The first point of ethics of the counsellor's professional code is: Even when the counsellor's personal value system is in conflict with that of the person being counselled, it is not for the counsellor to challenge the values of that person. Differ from, yes; challenge, no. If a strong conflict arises in the mind of the counsellor, it is better to excuse oneself from the case rather than work with a mind in turmoil.

The second, equally important ethical point is: Give the counselee the freedom to choose because eventually the consequences of that choice are lived by him. Never challenge the reality of the counselee. One can align the perception of realities through a change of perspective but never by confrontation. Therefore, it is required that the counsellor understand the point of view of the counselee.

Another major value the profession calls for is: Confidentiality of conversation and records is implicit, with no disclosure to anyone without the permission of the client. The only exception allowed is when one is dealing with a client of unsound mind and it makes sense for the wellbeing of the person to breach this cardinal principle.

Counsellors need to always remain on a learning path because the subject is vast. Be aware that 'I know that I know' is 5%; 'I know that I don't know' is another 5%; and 'I don't know that I don't know' is the remaining 90%.

Ethics of Counseellors

Counsellors should refrain from making their clients dependent on them. Setting them free to fly with the strength of their own wings, is the practice to follow. This is especially important as counsellors sometimes feel overcome when things do not work out well and the client does not make progress or stops coming for counselling, without any notice. We should remember we are not in the business of repairing the behaviour of all those who come to us. We sometimes succeed in helping people – and sometimes not. At the end of the day, it is a joint venture between two partners.

We counsellors have to remember it is not our job to teach morals to our clients. Morals are best left to men of religion. As mentioned earlier, our stance has to be non-judgmental while maintaining our principles and ethical code. Counsellors have to develop a professional attitude since the stress factors are high in this domain.

FALLING IN LOVE IN THERAPY: No....no
BEING LOVE IN THERAPY: YES...yes

Transference and counter-transference have been briefly discussed in earlier chapters. Transference is the feeling a patient has towards his counsellor and counter-transference is the opposite phenomenon. Whenever this subject is discussed, we counsellors are told to be aware of the feeling we have towards our clients and not to let these come in the way of therapy. Scott Peck rubbishes this philosophy. Most counselees have been denied love in their lives by their parents, spouses, colleagues, and their environment. It is a major cause of mental illness. They are seeking love but love and sexuality are perceived as two sides of the same coin. M. Scott Peck explains love in the context of therapy saying: 'First of all, the role of the good therapist is that of a good parent, and good parents do not consummate sexual relationships with their children for some very compelling reason. The job of the parent is to be of use to a child and not to use the child for personal satisfaction. The job of a therapist is to be of use to the client and not use the client for the therapist's own needs. The job of the parent is to move the child to independence and so is the job of the therapist.'

Ethics of Counseellors

The moment sexual feelings come in, objectivity disappears. Your own needs take priority over everything else. Scott Peck adds: 'Since genuine love demands respect for the separate identity of the beloved, the genuinely loving therapist will recognize and accept what the patient's paths in life is, and should be, separate from the therapist. Also the client comes to us travelling great distances to be with us and the client needs love and warmth in the session and not only intellectual conversation. It is through love and warmth that one stays on the journey of spiritual growth…. *A minimally trained lay therapist who exercises a great capacity to love will achieve psycho-therapeutic results that equal those of the very best psychiatrists.'*

OPENNESS TO CHALLENGE

For any permanent change to take place we must contemplate and be open to challenge and the biggest challenges that come to us are mostly from within us than outside of us. It is so much easier for us to examine the world outside of us than within us. It is a challenge for most of us but so much more for those who are going through emotional traumas. Finally, it has to be accepted that if we want to move from our current position to the desired position, we have to examine ourselves from within and challenge our currently held realities. If we don't do that, Dr. Peck explains that situation with a perfect analogy. This is what he says: "Otherwise we live in a closed system-within a bell jar, re-breathing our own fetid air, more and more subject to delusion."

I have mentioned already that about 20% of the people who come for counselling pull out by choice because they are not willing to re-examine their current position. For them, the pain of change is greater than remaining the same. Even those of us who consider ourselves mentally healthy, lack the will for internal re-examination, with the result that we realize only a small part of our total potential.

By going in for counselling, that act alone opens us to the deepest questions from counsellors. During the course of conversations with the therapist, insights are received about our lives, which are often

Ethics of Counseellors

contradictory to our current beliefs. That requires an attitude of openness to change in order to gain the fruits of that effort. The reason some of us do not reach out for counselling is not because we do not have the time but because we do not want our current beliefs and behaviour to come under scrutiny.

Dr. Peck brings out another point which the majority of us in the counselling field have experienced, not once but many times over – that many clients come to us with the impression the therapist has a quick-fix solution leading to immediate relief. After narrating their story, they ask for a simple, straightforward solution. They do not realize that any solution can at best be a band-aid that covers the grievous wound. The true healing has to come from within.

Another aspect of therapy M. Scott Peck brings out is that many clients spend time narrating superficial and peripheral issues rather than the real ones confronting them.

There is yet another category of people who come for counselling – those who want tips on how to change the behaviour of others. For example: 'I am having an issue with my wife which is causing disturbance in my married life. Can you give me a solution to change how my wife behaves?' Or 'My son has become wayward. How can I correct his behaviour?' Such clients do not realize that they themselves have to pick the ball and play and not keep bouncing it back to others.

The following representative statement narrative shows the games people can play in disowning personal responsibility: 'We have done everything possible for our boy. We have even gone to four different counsellors with him. But nothing has helped.'

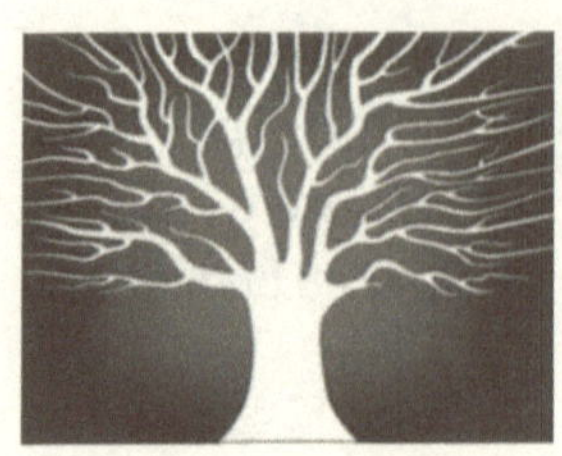

Part III: Mental Conditions
An overview

I hated being depressed, but it was also in depression that I learned my own acreage, the full extent of my soul. ~ Andrew Solomon

I mentioned right in the beginning that my beacon, my Guru, in psychotherapy, is M. Scott Peck, author of the bestselling book, *The Road Less Travelled.* In the spiritual realm gurus such as Meher Baba and Sai Shridi Baba have been great teachers with massive followings; but for me, Dr. Peck is the greatest teacher of all. What follows is a brief chapter culled from his writings. Here, I am no more than a conduit for his teaching. Anyone wishing to progress in the domain of counselling, will benefit tremendously from the perusal of his books. He demystifies many myths using only a scientific temper.

Mental illnesses

Although this part of the book is no more than a few thousand words, the subject falls into a different area which strictly belongs to professionals in the field of psychiatry, a domain counsellors support with their work. To use a *filmi* metaphor – here, the psychiatrists are the heroes or main actors and the counsellors are the supporting cast. This section deals with mental illnesses and is most relevant for caregivers, who need to be able to detect signs of mental illness in the early stages and seek help, before the issues get consolidated and embedded. If caregivers have doubts about where to seek help, counsellors can guide them in the relevant direction. But seeking help is a must because the problem will not dissolve by itself.

I begin with the disclaimer that I am a lay counsellor and not a psychiatrist or specialist in this domain. I simply share some basic facts we need to know about mental illnesses in order to underline the difference between mental sprains (emotional issues brought out in the various case studies in this book), and mental fractures (cases of mental illnesses which need referral to specialists). What has been covered thus far is what lay counsellors or therapists can take care of. In counselling terms, these issues are often referred to as Transient Situational Disturbances (TSDs) – as in the case studies discussed in Part I. In this chapter, we deal with mental conditions that clearly fall outside the domain of lay counselling. However, counsellors do need to have a basic knowledge and awareness of mental illnesses as well. This enables them to identify and refer such cases to psychiatrists. It also helps counsellors support the family in dealing with the stress of living with a mentally ill person. Mentally ill people inevitably take the whole family on a stressful journey and it is important they too, seek counselling to retain their composure and deal with the stress.

MANIC DEPRESSION

One day, a client was brought to me by his wife. This is what she had to tell me: Her husband had been behaving erratically for a couple of years. He would make embarrassing remarks in company; so much so, she had to stop socialising in order to avoid his 'uncouth behaviour'. Over time, she had learnt to cope. However, what she could not cope with were the recent changes in him. He went on buying sprees without a care in the world. He would buy fifty CDs at one go, DVDs by the dozen, neckties, cufflinks and watches, which he never wore; order books on Amazon on his credit card; and give expensive gifts to friends and family. Their finances were in disarray. He was not in touch with reality. Yet he was full of energy and could do with little sleep. Sometimes, he would make inappropriate and sexually explicit remarks in the presence of young people.

Then, while she was struggling with this behaviour, he swung to the other extreme and became exactly the opposite. He sat switching from one TV channel to another, he could not concentrate. He seemed listless, would get up very late, and had lost interest in personal hygiene. He avoided contact with people and would respond to all conversations in monosyllables. His food habits had become erratic, and he would blame her and the children for what was happening to him.

When I had spent some time with the client, it became clear he was suffering from manic depression. His mood swings said it all. In such cases, the counsellor has to use all the soft skills at his command to persuade the patient and family to see a psychiatrist. The very mention of the word tends to raise their hackles. 'Are you saying my husband has gone mad?' is a common demand. A plea like: 'I am sure *you* can handle it, Sir,' is another response. A counsellor must be ready to spend time and energy to convince clients it is in their best interests to seek medical intervention. It must be done. Often, I have had to say I would be happy to continue seeing the patient while he was under medication, but without that step, I could not. Do clients need the parallel intervention of counsellors and doctors? I believe they do. With so few doctors working in this field, they simply do not have the time to counsel patients and their families.

Psychosis and Neurosis

The best explanation to highlight the difference between these two illnesses is, a psychotic grandly declares he is Mahatma Gandhi while the neurotic meekly wishes he was Mahatma Gandhi.

Let us discuss psychosis first. A person who truly believes he is Mahatma Gandhi is not likely to seek help because he does not believe there is anything the matter with him. He is convinced it would be better for the world to believe his identity. Logic and rationality also goes overboard when the person believes he has acquired superhuman ability. I know of no easy way to deal with such a maladjusted personality except to advise their near and dear ones to seek the help of mental health organisations as soon as they see such delusionary behaviour.

Neurosis, on the other hand, is a case of excessive and disproportionate reaction. Most of us have a healthy fear of danger but if such fears lock a person into a shell, it becomes neurotic anxiety. Something that needs to be stated upfront is that such fears should not be ignored or made little of. If you insist such fears are unrealistic, you may be putting the person in danger. You may know mothers who stand in front of the gate at home because the child is ten minutes late returning from school. They keep looking at their watches and saying , 'I don't know what has happened. I don't know why the bus is so late.' This can broadly be termed anxiety neurosis.

Then there are those amongst us who climb seven floors of a hotel to reach their rooms because they have a lift phobia. You would also have heard of hypochondriacs who imagine they suffer from all kinds of illnesses. Even when they have been cleared by doctors, they self-medicate. These cases too, need medical intervention. Doctors play the lead roles and counsellors are the supporting cast.

PASSIVE AGGRESSIVE

You too, will have met people in your family or organisation, who do not oppose any idea being discussed. They give the impression that the decisions being taken are in sync with their thoughts; but the moment they are on their own, they do everything to ensure the ideas fail. Let me illustrate with an organizational example. Assume a decision is taken by the boss, in consultation with the group, that a particular supplier should be given preference because of the quality of his product. However, the passive aggressive believes otherwise. Such a person will quietly go about making the decision fail. He is aggressive, but in a passive way.

This is the first stage. Since they do not say anything openly and nod at every suggestion, passive aggressive people are not easy to understand. You cannot reach them and it is very difficult to relate to them. In the process, they irritate and anger others, in much the same way as openly aggressive people do. They find ways to delay; they forget to pay back loans; and if any demands are made of them, get ready to be blackmailed. Avoidance is the best policy in such cases. As a counsellor, I do not get involved with passive aggressive. In one such case I was threatened that if I did not do what the person wanted, he would 'take care of me'.

Narcissistic personality characteristic

'Self-absorbed' is another description for narcissists. Being full of themselves, as if the whole world revolves around them, is their characteristic. If the world refuses to revolve around them, they get angry. Some amount of narcissism is present in each of us but when it becomes all-pervasive and goes beyond self-esteem and the person begins to think that others are mere extensions of himself, he becomes narcissistic. In extreme cases, it can turn malignant and a narcissist can harm others. We often submit to the will of others or say it is God's will. But people afflicted with malignant narcissism do not believe in the will of God. There is no higher power for them. In extreme cases, they can be evil. When they reach that stage, their acts become destructive. They cannot take any criticism and are capable of causing harm. They are pretentious and their public image is very important to them. Even when they are vengeful and hurtful, they deny acting that way. Narcissists can be very devious people. The best way is to disengage from them and stay out of their way.

Personality adaptations: Do you know who you are?

As I come to the end of this book, here is a quiz to solve. It is titled, 'Do you know who you are?' As mentioned before, there are many approaches to counselling. Transactional Analysis (TA) is one of them. In the framework of reference of TA teachings, it is believed that each of us fits into a psychological box or a fix – by and large, that is. You will have other personality traits but your centre of gravity will revolve around one box. Now we come to the quiz. Which of the states or adaptations (from the first column) mentioned below, best describes you?

An Overview

Adaptation	Characteristics	Description	Drivers	Injunctions
Schizoid	Withdrawn passivity, day dreaming, avoidance	Shy, overly sensitive, eccentric	Be strong, try hard to please others	Don't make it, don't belong here, don't enjoy, don't be sane, don't think, don't feel (love, sex, joy)
Hysterical	Excitability, emotional instability, over reactivity, dramatic, attention getting, seductive	Immature, self-centred, vain, dependant	Please me, try hard, hurry up	Don't grow up, don't be important, don't think
Paranoid	Rigidity of thoughts, grandiosity, projection	Hypersensitive, suspicious, jealous, envious	Be strong, be perfect	Don't be a child, don't feel, don't be close, don't enjoy
Antisocial	Conflict with society, low frustration, tolerance, need for excitement and drama	Selfish, suspicious, jealous, envious	Be strong, please others	Don't feel, don't be close, don't enjoy
Passive aggressive	Aggression, resentment	Obstructive, stubborn	Try harder, be strong	Don't feel, don't be close, don't enjoy, don't make it
Obsessive compulsive	Conformity, Conscientious-ness	Perfectionist, overly inhibited, overly conscientious, overly dutiful, tense	Be strong, be perfect	Don't be a child, don't feel, don't be close, don't enjoy

An Overview

Drivers are messages taken in by the child from authority figures at post verbal stage. Injunctions are messages taken by the child in preverbal stage. My wife and I did the adaptation test and she concluded that she did not fit into any of the boxes. I concluded that I came close to the Obsessive Compulsive box. Have you figured out your psychological box? Neither this nor that? A bit of everything? Don't worry – these are just rough guidelines. I mentioned this at the beginning of the chapter but it bears repetition – those afflicted with any of the mental illnesses dealt with here, will not notice anything abnormal about themselves. It is important for family and friends to observe abnormalities and seek out help.

There are two ways to seek help. One is to go to the nearest counselling centre and ask for guidance. Most centres have websites and can be found by surfing the internet. The second way is to seek help from a psychiatrist. I recommend the first option for the simple reason that the family also needs counselling help because living with such people can be highly stressful. They leave things unfinished. They do not turn up for meetings on time because they have something else to do. They hurt others. They never climb the ladder of success through teamwork. The only time they react is when they are being fired by the boss or disengaged by the family. I have had zero success with this type of disorder, despite reaching out, understanding, challenging or hurting to heal. In such cases I tell the family I am unable to help the person and the choice then lies with them to find an alternative counsellor or a doctor.

OBSESSIVE COMPULSIVE DISORDER (OCD)

To describe it in simple terms, 'obsessive' relates to recurring thoughts. Even when the person wants to chase them out of their minds, the thoughts persist. They persist even if he does not want to act on them. 'Compulsive' relates to the overpowering need to perform an act(s). Compulsion can lead to acting on thoughts like rearranging the room or desk, putting everything in place, and having a kind of compulsory order in life. Checking repeatedly to ensure the geyser has been switched off or the room locked, washing hands frequently, rigidity in actions, the my-way-or-the-highway approach to living, are some other signs. People with this condition resent others controlling them.

Counselling requires emotional contact and psychological bonding with clients to understand their feelings. Those with OCD, on the other hand, avoid closeness. They do everything to dissipate it. For this reason, it is best to deal with them intellectually through discussions and hope to glide in an insight that appeals to their frame of reference. Counsellors and family have to remember such a person will cause them stress, hence it is wise to remain alert on that front. It is quite likely that one will get an impression that no headway is being made through counselling, despite intellectual inputs and persuasions. I find it best to let people with OCD explain their positions and hope that though their own words, they will gain some insights which they will want to work with. Tap into them for them to tap themselves.

SCHIZOPHRENIA

A simply understood word for this is 'insanity'. In such people, there is a complete disintegration of personality. What schizophrenics think, do and feel, are incongruent. They suffer from delusions and can think they are the creators of this planet. If they happen to see some powdery substance lying around, they imagine someone is planning to poison them. One person told me his ex-boss (who had not been in contact with him for the last 20 years), had hired people to follow him on bikes. He truly believed a serious plot was being hatched against him. Hearing voices in the mind or voices giving instructions, is another symptom. Schizophrenics need to be taken to a psychiatrist immediately. This is not a condition that can be overcome by will power or personal resolve. Nor can the family take care of such a person. Medical help is essential to lead these tormented people to a place of peace.

ANTISOCIAL PERSONALITIES

Also termed psychopaths, these people are strangely perverted. They persistently and compulsively violate laws, commit offences, steal, cheat and lie. At the same time they try to talk their way out of difficult or incriminating situations. They harm others without any remorse. Devoid of principles, they act in any way which attains their ends. They have no sense of right and wrong.

These are just some of the many kinds of mental illnesses we humans beings are prone to. While some may be the result of childhood or adult traumas, others are conditions over which the individual has no control. But no matter what the case may be, each of these mental disorders requires the help of a specialist. Many people do overcome their conditions to get a fresh lease on life. Counsellors are cautioned not to label any of these disorders, as they are not equipped to do so.

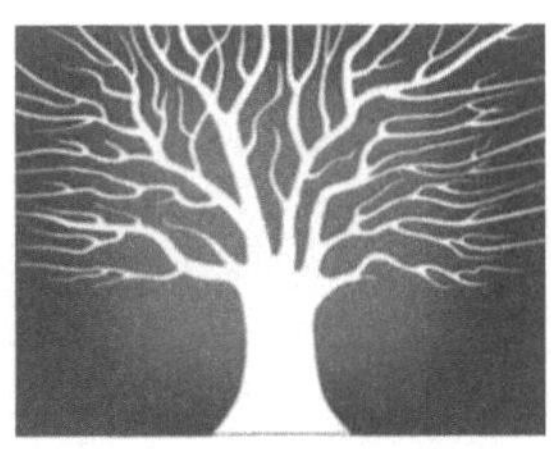 Empathy, the Power Within

If there is one attribute, just one attribute, the counsellor must possess, it is empathy. Ched Meng Tan, author of *Search Inside Yourself,* recommends the following, to help develop this critical quality.

Just Like Me & Loving Kindness Meditation
Sit in a comfortable position which allows you to be alert and relaxed at the same time. Start with 2 minutes to rest the mind on the breath. Bring to mind someone you care about. Visualise him or her. If you wish, use a photograph or video of the person. Now read the script slowly to yourself, pausing at the end of each sentence as reflection:

Just Like me
This person has a body and a mind, just like me.
This person has feelings, emotions, and thoughts just like me.
This person has, at some point of time in his her life, been sad and disappointed, angry, hurt, or confused, just like me.
This person wishes to be free from pain and suffering, just like me.
This person wishes to be healthy and loved, and to have fulfilling relationship, just like me
This person wishes to be happy, just like me

Now, allow some wishes to arise.
Loving Kindness
I wish this person to have strength, the resources, and the emotional and social support to navigate the difficulties in life.
I wish this person to be free from pain and suffering.
I wish this person to be happy
Because, this person is fellow human being just like me (pause)
Now, I wish for everybody I know to be happy (long pause)

End with 1 minute of resting the mind.

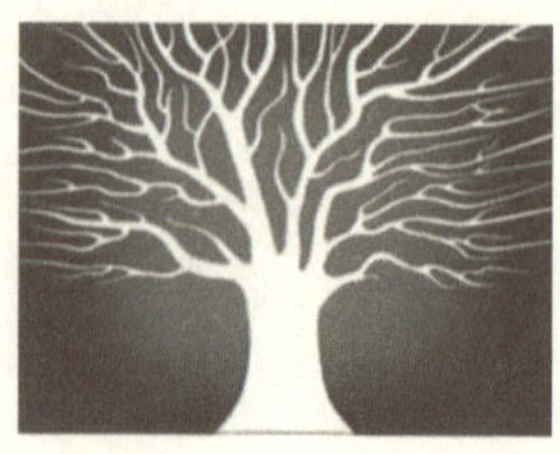

Love, joy, and peace cannot flourish until you have freed yourself from mind dominance. ~ Eckhart Tolle

As mentioned at the beginning of the book, understanding of mental health issues in Indian society is woefully inadequate. It still remains a little known fact that most mental issues can be effectively handled with the guidance of a lay councellor – only the most severe cases need to be referred to a specialist. It is long overdue that the subject of mental health no longer remains confined to professionals, but is brought out into the open and discussed in a language that every person understands. An American friend of mine sometimes interrupts our long-distance calls to say she has an appointment with her 'shrink' and therefore has to sign off. But in India, it is rare for even the most educated amongst us, to so much as mention the state of our mental health.

The idea of this book is to bring mental health issues on a common platform where they belong; and in some small way, address the skewed emphasis towards physical health. For any human being to be healthy, a balance of mind and body is not only necessary but imperative.

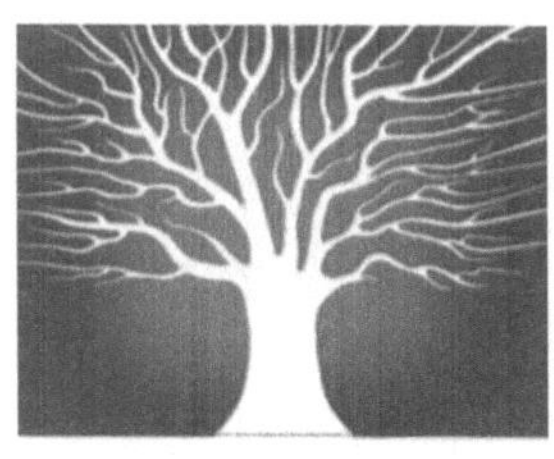

SANJIVINI SOCIETY FOR MENTAL HEALTH

A - 6, Satsang Vihar Marg
Qutab Institutional Area, New Delhi 110067
Phone : 011 26862222 /26864488
Email : directorsanjivinisociety@gmail.com
Website : www.sanjivinisociety.org

SUMAITRI

Aradhana Hostel Complex, Basement no. 1
Bhagwan Das Road, New Delhi 110001
Phone : 011 23389090
Website : www.sumaitri.org

VISHWAS SOCIETY FOR MENTAL HEALTH

Suraj Plaza, 203, second floor
8th F main Road, Jayanagar 3rd Block
Bangalore 560 011, Karnataka
Email: Vishwascounselling.org
Website: Vishwas.bangalore@yahoo.com

SNEHA COUNSELLING CENTRE

Hymamshu Jyothi Kala Peetha
4th Main Road, 17th Cross
Malleswaram, Bangalore 560055
Phone : +91 9342505975, +91 9342133520
Email: snehacounselling@yahoo.com
Website snehacounselling.org

Select List of Counselling Centres

VIVEKA CENTRE FOR EMOTIONAL SUPPORT
Viveka Trust
#3271, First Floor, 11th Main
HAL 2nd Stage, Indiranagar,
Bangalore 560 008, Karnataka
Phone: +91-80-6533 0387
e-mail: support@vivekatrust
http://www.vivekatrust.org/about-us.php

HELPING HAND
Banjara Academy
418, Ist Main Ist Block, RT Nagar
Bangalore 560 032, Karnataka
 Phone: 080 23535787, 23535766
Mobile: +91 9342472305
Website www.banjaraacademy.org

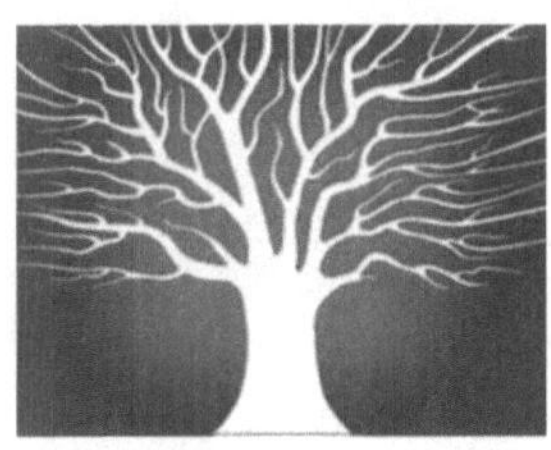

1. *A Handbook for Lay Counsellors*

2. Carkhuff, Rober R. *The Art of Helping*

3. Cully, Sue. *Integrative counselling skills in action*

4. Currie, Fr. Joe. S J. *Barefoot Counsellor*

5. Ibid. *In the path of the Barefoot Counsellor*

6. Glasser, William. *Choice Theory*

7. Hicks, James Whitney MD. *50 Signs Of Mental Illness*

8. Jones, Richard. *Practical Counselling and Helping Skills*

9. Kennedy, Eugene & Sara Charles MD. *ON Becoming a Counsellor*

10. Peck, M. Scott. *The Road less Travelled*

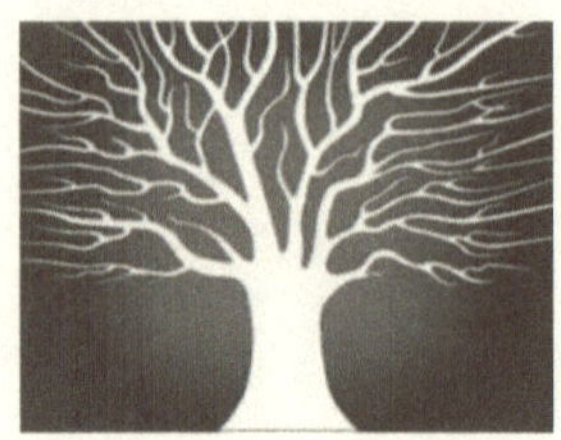

Acknowledgements

I am deeply grateful for the help received from Sonya Kaushik, in editing the first draft, and Maya Jayapal, author and counsellor, for her encouragement all through the process of writing.

www.ingramcontent.com/pod-product-compliance
Lightning Source LLC
Chambersburg PA
CBHW051257250726
48656CB00004B/1343